DISABILITY AND MANAGED CARE

DISABILITY AND MANAGED CARE

Problems and Opportunities at the End of the Century

ARNOLD BIRENBAUM

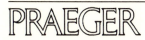

Westport, Connecticut
London

Library of Congress Cataloging-in-Publication Data

Birenbaum, Arnold.
   Disability and managed care : problems and opportunities at the
end of the century / Arnold Birenbaum.
      p.   cm.
   Includes bibliographical references and index.
   ISBN 0–275–96552–X (alk. paper)
   1. Managed care plans (Medical care)—United States.
   2. Handicapped—Medical care—United States.   I. Title.
   RA413.5.U5B494   1999
   362.1′04258′0973—dc21   99–23415

British Library Cataloguing in Publication Data is available.

Library of Congress Catalog Card Number: 99–23415
ISBN: 0–275–96552–X

First published in 1999

Praeger Publishers, 88 Post Road West, Westport, CT 06881
An imprint of Greenwood Publishing Group, Inc.
www.praeger.com

Printed in the United States of America

The paper used in this book complies with the
Permanent Paper Standard issued by the National
Information Standards Organization (Z39.48–1984).

10 9 8 7 6 5 4 3 2 1

Contents

Preface

During the past decade the community of those with disabilities has emerged as a distinctive political force in American life. The passage in 1990 of the Americans with Disabilities Act marks the recognition of accommodations to people with disabilities as part of their civil rights. Disability is no longer seen as something to hide; nor should people with disabilities live lives of isolation and understimulation. More and more people are seeing themselves and are seen by others as having a condition that limits their capacity to pursue major life activities. Consequently, there is a greater demand today to find better ways to live with disabilities, including, for example, home modifications, assistive technology, and access to high quality medical care. These interventions often can increase an individual's productivity by: reducing the number of days when he or she cannot perform full-time social roles (e.g., work, school); allowing for more independence; and improving the person's capacity to be included in ordinary activities in the community.

Health care, however, has undergone a serious revolution that threatens some of these goals and objectives. We are dealing with the consequences of that revolution as consumers and as providers of health care. Despite these vast changes, access to quality care at reasonable cost is not guaranteed for all Americans. Since the failure of health care reform in 1994, more Americans than ever before are without health insurance. Even when employers offer health insurance and pay half the costs, many workers find the cost of insurance unaffordable.

Spokespeople for the managed care industry argue that it is only managed care that will create affordable health care for all in the United States. Market forces have led the charge toward the conversion of health insurance from indemnity coverage to cost-driven managed care in its many manifestations. State and federally funded programs such as Medicaid and Medicare are also seeking out the presumed cost-containment benefits of managed care. To what extent is a system of health care, both privately and publicly financed, that is moving toward both explicit and implicit rationing of care able to meet the ongoing needs of people with disabilities? The chapters that follow will attempt to answer this question.

I sought in this endeavor to encompass all of the disability and health policy issues that are being generated, as the system evolves. I have, perhaps, relied disproportionately on studies related to developmental disabilities to create a picture of the major changes and consequences for individuals and institutions. Given my career experiences as a medical sociologist and health policy analyst concerned with developmental disabilities, this is understandable. I am seeking to look to the past, the present, and the future.

Even the generalizations in the following pages about managed care may not hold forever. In the language of economics, in many metropolitan regions, the system is moving toward high market penetration by managed care and maturing markets, with a small number of plans covering large numbers of lives.

On a national scale, the health care system is losing its excess capacity. The implications of provider downsizing and the reconfiguration of medical procedures, following clinical practice guidelines, is of major focus in the pages that follow. In this book I have dealt with the consequences of managed care in all of its facets for people with disabilities. This analysis identifies the structural advantages and disadvantages of managed care for people with disabilities. Within this discussion, for example, I examine the extent to which new or experimental procedures are not paid for by managed care plans.

As has been suggested by disability advocates, when it comes to evaluating whether the managed care revolution is a good thing, the disabled are like canaries in the mines. The inference is that the disabled are stand-ins for us all. Their fate should be of great interest to others who might also suffer from cost containment. As the saying goes, we may all be only a stop sign away from being disabled.

The subject of disability and social change is one that I have researched, written about, and even taught to graduate students. Much of my career as a sociologist and a health policy analyst has been built around these studies and linked to agencies that delivered services in the community. In the 1960s, I evaluated a major project that integrated recreational groups for mentally retarded adults and adolescents in community centers, YW/MCAs, and settlement houses. I also studied in detail the role conceptions and performances of mothers of mentally retarded children.

In the 1970s, I studied efforts to resettle former adult state school residents who had been placed there as children because their parents had been told that individuals with mental retardation belonged in large and isolated facilities. As I followed some of these individuals out of a community residence to smaller living arrangements, I continued to monitor the implementation of state and national policy to close institutions and asylums and create community living. In the 1980s, I studied the utilization of medical care, its financing, and its cost for children, adolescents and adults with severe developmental disabilities.

At the same time, I followed closely the dynamics of health care in the United States, including the concern about the overtreatment of patients in the fee-for-service system, a consequence of the low level of accountability of physicians. Through field observations and classroom teaching I also acquired an interest in the development of new and changing professions in the health care field. I studied and wrote about the development of new primary care roles through the use of advanced practice nurses and the effort to transform the profession of pharmacy from medication provider to clinical consultant on how to use drugs safely and how to promote patient adherence.

I have never attempted to be a narrow specialist. Nor have I dismissed the value of in-depth specialization to analyze complex subjects. I have sought to be scholarly but am aware of the importance of seeing the larger picture, the forest and the trees. Through these attempts to synthesize a great deal of knowledge, I was able to learn much about the way in which Americans receive care and pay for it, and what the eventual costs are for health care services. I have been fortunate in that I could integrate my general interests in the American health care system at large with my special interest in the social consequences of disability.

While my career as a medical sociologist and health policy analyst may not be as long as, let us say, baseball pitcher Gaylord Perry's, nor as controversial, I do believe I have contributed to the public dialogue on two important issues: (1) how we can have a quality health care system at reasonable cost that serves all Americans and (2) disability and health care. For the latter subject, I also pose the generic question, how do people with disabilities deal with the social institutions that are their sources of help and sometimes despair?

This book hopefully will contribute to that same public dialogue and offer a way to understand managed care from the perspectives of consumers and providers. It is largely a "report card" concerning the issue of how this vast change in health care, organization, delivery and financing impacts on people with disabilities.

Bronx, New York, 1999

Acknowledgments

My longstanding involvement in the field of disability and health policy is built on working relationships with a number of individuals. For this book, I collaborated with Herbert J. Cohen, M.D., on the analysis of the data collected from programs on the impact of managed care on their services, training programs, and other functions. We also worked together on a national survey of state maternal and child health programs and how they were responding to managed care. Herb and I have worked together on many research projects and policy analyses, going back over a quarter century. A longtime developmental pediatrician and advocate in the field of developmental disabilities, he continues to be a source of sage advice, as well as one of the most politically astute players in the world of disability.

Bob Griss, Director of the Center on Disability and Health in Washington, D.C., is a most demanding advocate as well as a visionary in the field of disability. His tightly reasoned policy papers provided guidance in the development of the manuscript. Our long phone conversations, interrupted by occasional but wonderful face-to-face discussions, provided challenging problems that I had to solve in writing these chapters. For the past two years, Bob was my "generalized other": I often wondered in writing, what would Bob think of this insight or presentation?

Bob also provided me with an intellectual network to help improve the range of discussion on measuring disability and opportunities to learn more about the health consequences of physical disabilities. Through the Center on Disability and Health, I encountered a senior health policy advisor, and a new mentor, Ray Seltser, M.D., Dean Emeritus and Professor of Epidemiology Emeritus at the University of Pittsburgh Graduate School of Public Health. Dr. Seltser graciously read the entire manuscript. His constructive comments motivated me to research and write some important additions to the work, particularly in chapter 4.

Support staff at the Rose F. Kennedy University Affiliated Program for People with Developmental Disabilities, Albert Einstein College of Medicine, gave generously of their time to find reference material and encouragement. In particular, Roberta Ippolito, Michele Soanes, and Sophie Walsh were extremely helpful and there when I needed them.

Funding for these surveys, studies, and analyses came, in part, from the core grant to the Rose F. Kennedy University Affiliated Program for People with Developmental Disabilities from the Administration on Developmental Disabilities, Administration on Children and Families, and from the Leadership in Education in Neurologic Diseases training grant from the Maternal and Child Health Bureau, Health Resources Services Agency. Both agencies are part of the United States Department of Health and Human Services.

Introduction

When patients present symptoms to physicians, it is often in the form of a story about their findings, feelings, and failings related to their bodies. Personal stories help us understand society and its institutions, as well. A great deal of anger, bitterness, and resentment is expressed when people with serious chronic illnesses and disabilities analyze the profession of medicine, or if you prefer, the broader health care system. Other emotions are also expressed. Relationships matter, even when the two partners of the relationship are unequal. A bond sometimes exists between people with disabilities and the professionals who assist them. This bond is illustrated by the flip comments made by adolescents with spina bifida who refer to the surgeons who have operated on them so many times and have discussed them so often at professional meetings that they are not just their doctors but their agents. The wry humor manifest in this observation reflects the structured ambivalence in the relationship.

Doctors can do more sometimes than attempt to fix a body that does not work. Born mute and paralyzed, Christopher Nolan became an award-winning Irish poet. There was no miracle cure for Nolan. In his autobiographical essay, *Under the Eye of the Clock* (1987), he tells how a Fitzwilliam Street, Dublin doctor, in an almost life-bestowing way, identified a core of intelligence and personality in him—a 17 month old severely disabled by cerebral palsy:

Watching and listening, the blue-eyed doctor heard of a mother's quiet observations of her son. . . . Assessing him, the doctor wisely played games with
the child. He blew into his eyes once but when Joseph heard him taking a
deep breath he was ready for him and cutely closed his eyes. Then when the
doctor failed to blow the boy opened his eyes to see what was wrong. (51)

What followed from this simple confirmation of normal intelligence was a
prescription for physiotherapy, speech therapy, occupational therapy, and
most important, schooling. Stimulation was necessary to foster the development of the self locked inside a body that did not work.

Clearly, Nolan's words capture an event where his potential for growth
was found. Moreover, as a writer, Nolan's extraordinary accomplishment is
that he adumbrates his difficulties lyrically and never evokes pity. The
warmth and intelligence of his family comes shining through. In contrast,
autobiographical descriptions of disabilities acquired later in life present a
picture of lost selves, a diminution of status, and unwanted dependencies.
When the body fails to work there is a loss of identity.

The language of the social sciences contrasts sharply with Nolan's poeti-
cal expressions. The American anthropologist Robert F. Murphy (1987)
describes the acquisition of his major disability in midlife as shaping his
sense of self and identity in a far stronger way than anything related to age,
work, or ethnicity. Disability, in the language of sociology, is a master status.

The presence of a disability dominates Murphy's life in all of its facets,
throughout his waking hours and even his dreams. In a more refined sense,
disability represents limits on his presentation of self. Murphy's ability to
compartmentalize his life among different audiences was eliminated when
he became first a paraplegic and then a quadriplegic. Moreover, the actor-
as-cripple is subject to a great deal of scrutiny by others.

A serious disability inundates all other claims to social standing, relegating
to secondary status all the attainments of life, all other social roles, even
sexuality. It is not a role; it is an identity, a dominant characteristic to which
all social roles must be adjusted. (106)

Despite the continuous reminders of his new identity, reinforced in public by his dependence on a wheelchair, Murphy admits he could not survive
without assistance. He becomes part of the world of rehabilitation medicine, much like an object to be tinkered with, and he dissociates his body
from his self: "The paralytic becomes accustomed to being lifted, rolled,
pushed, pulled, and twisted, and he survives this treatment by putting emotional distance between himself and his body" (100–101).

Access to services was probably not an issue when Murphy became disabled. Now the services received by people with disabilities are subject to new and recurrent reviews and authorizations that are part of the conversion from fee-for-service medicine to managed care. There have also been changes initiated in medical practice styles, given the goal of cost cutting that has come into our lives along with managed care. The issue has been raised by self-advocating people with disabilities and others that this new form of delivery of health care services will limit their access to what they need. A 1998 national survey of people with disabilities, commissioned by the private nonprofit National Organization on Disability, found a slightly increasing minority from four years ago—21 percent—saying they did not receive the medical care they needed on at least one occasion in the past year. In contrast, only 11 percent of a random sample of people without disabilities had the same experience in 1998 (National Organization on Disability, 1998: 6).

Today there is an obvious connection between the human experience of acquiring and living with a disability and the market forces that have swept away many of the conventions and practices found in the traditional American health care system. At one time the experience of disability might be characterized exclusively by isolation and loneliness. This is hardly the case today as people with disabilities write about their experiences and lead lives where risk taking occurs in public discourse and public places. The movement has created much greater political and cultural sensitivity to issues that impact on the disabled.

The success of the disability movement has endowed with a new meaning the following comments by the great American sociologist and social critic, C. Wright Mills. Writing in *The Sociological Imagination* in 1959, Mills saw the importance of being conscious of one's life in a social environment that permitted communications with others in the same situation:

> The individual can understand his own experience and gauge his fate by locating himself within his period. . . . He can know his own chances in life only by becoming aware of those of all individuals in his circumstances. (5)

Despite the successes of the disability movement to organize and articulate its point of view, there are vast changes in the American health care system that make the experience of heavy users of the system relevant, not just to people with disabilities, but to all members of this society. People with disabilities are proxies for everyone else. For most of us, particularly those under 60, contacts with health care providers are infrequent, and we receive direct services from a limited number of experts. However, this is only the visible part of a social institution. As a complex set of arrangements designed to meet human needs, the health care system is part of our commercial life, our state and national governments, and our relationship with our employers. Many of these arrangements have remained hidden from most Americans, although the part that was hidden—how health care was paid for and who paid—has become the focal point of much discussion and concern. This has happened because managed care is seen as limiting access to needed services and not just as a way of saving money. The administrators of such systems of care are now regarded by many Americans as uncaring. Many of us worry whether complex medical care will be there when we need it.

Consider how the shift of focus among analysts and critics of how the health care system is organized has changed decisively in less than two decades. In 1981 I wrote, with some justification, that

> the common experience of going to the doctor and paying the bills has recently left many Americans wondering about whether services are for the benefit of the patients or for those who seek to heal them, operate hospitals or manufacture and distribute pharmaceuticals. (Birenbaum, 1981: 1)

As we near the beginning of a new millennium, we would probably substitute health maintenance organizations (HMO) for the litany of providers and manufacturers, seen as exploitative, found in the second part of the sentence. Ironically, providers and manufacturers today would probably join their fellow Americans in wondering whether they will survive in the future, given the cost-cutting thrusts of managed care.

It is not only the providers and patients who are struck by the difference between the way things were under indemnity health insurance and under the new type of insurance providers. Some executives of the insurance companies and the providers they paid are also feeling that there is a change in corporate culture being brought about through the triumph of managed care.

Aetna Inc., an old-line health insurance company, acquired the brash U.S. Healthcare, a tough HMO with an aggressive style toward demanding deep discounts from providers. After the acquisition in July 1996, the top management of Aetna sought to integrate U.S. Healthcare's senior executives into the top positions in the new corporation.

As reporter Lucette Lagnado (1998) notes, the change has lost Aetna many friends:

> Two years later, the merger, while invigorating Aetna in some ways has cost it dearly in others. Numerous patients, employers and doctors have been unnerved by the company's sharp shifts. Aetna once paid claims promptly and with little question; now it is prone to mishandling charges, pays far less for

the same services and sometimes keeps doctors waiting months before settling their bills. . . .

In the ensuing backlash, hundreds of doctors have dropped out. Aetna says that overall, its doctor ranks are growing steadily. But in certain areas, many have defected. . . . In Dallas, Aetna faced the loss of a group of 500 physicians. It is trying to woo them back one by one. (A1)

The quest for economic success in the highly competitive mature marketplaces, such as California, permeates the medical practice groups that contract with health maintenance organizations. Dr. Thomas W. Self, a pediatric gastroenterologist in San Diego, was forced to leave his medical group because his practice style was not compatible with the new culture of managed care. He was terminated, went to trial, and under the California Business and Professional Code, was found to be wrongfully dismissed and awarded defamation damages. Here is what Self faced as a practitioner:

Before the advent of managed care, I had a reputation for being a thorough and careful diagnostician. But as managed care became more powerful and as patients were turned into "cost units," my medical group, now affiliated with various H.M.O.'s, began to criticize my thoroughness as amounting to "overtesting," insecurity or indecisiveness. The board expressed concern that I would jeopardize future referrals to the group by managed care organizations, which were concerned with keeping costs down. (1998: A17)

People with disabilities deal with the new realities of health care financing and organization more frequently than those without disability. There is much to be learned from their experiences with managed care. They can provide us with insights into how their human spirits prevail, despite their private troubles. Through their experiences with the health care system, they can also reveal what needs to be fixed in managed care. It is important and useful to build on these experiences and insights from them, although I have more to say about the organization, financing, and delivery of health care under managed care than about specific results for individuals.

Chapter 1 begins from an interactionist perspective, as presented in a discussion of the social significance of discrepant identities. A heavy debt to the brilliant sociology of Erving Goffman is noted. Then the social origins and the political and economic consequences of disability are discussed. Efforts to determine the number of people in the population with disabilities are reviewed. A definition of disability is borrowed from the sociologist Gary Albrecht in order to shift the focus a bit from changing social and personal identities to the validation of disability to approve "safety-net" benefits and rehabilitation services.

Chapter 2 links people with disabilities to the health care system. It extends the discussion of the rates of utilization of medical care by people with disabilities in the United States, along with how that care is financed. Variations occur in the rates of utilization according to age and whether the person has insurance. The specific laws created to assist this sector of the population are identified.

The question of what is managed care is answered in chapter 3. The specific elements that are put in place in managed care organizations to deliver health care at lower costs are identified. The various models of organizing medical practice under managed care are discussed. In most managed care settings, the primary care providers are designated as the front line performers of service. They are gatekeepers to specialty care and to diagnostic testing. Incentives are established in these settings to get providers to initiate preventive interventions and early detections. In turn, there are incentives to husband scarce resources. The reasons why managed care and its cost-cutting features became attractive to benefits officers in corporations and the managers of Medicare and Medicaid, the two major publicly financed health insurance programs, are presented as part of the recent social history of the United States.

The gains and losses associated with a cost-driven health care system and how people with disabilities will fare under these conditions are addressed in chapter 4. It is clear that disability advocates and policy makers in the early 1990s became aware of managed care as a threat to accessing needed services. They worried more about stinting on services in managed care than the impact on people with disabilities of not having health insurance or having heavy out-of-pocket expenditures.

In chapter 5, I present information and analyze the situation of people with disabilities who are seeking to continue their access to specialists. With the trends for increased enrollment in managed care organizations, which will mean that more and more people with disabilities will be joining HMOs, it is to the advantage of these organizations to get ready for their new patients. This may involve training physicians to get them oriented to how to provide care for a person with a disability, including advocating for the person, when to say no to a patient who does not warrant further medical interventions, and how to develop the conceptual skill to determine when to continue to refer clients to specialists.

Chapter 6 discusses the two strands of concern with quality, the first of which is written into federal law to effect nondiscrimination. The goal of nondiscrimination was to make it possible for individuals with disabilities to find competitive employment, live independently, and enjoy benefits of community living in a manner similar to that of other citizens. As an unintended consequence, quality-of-life moved to the forefront of concern among disability advocates. The second quality issue has to do with the way managed care organizations have sought to prove that the care they give is as good or better than that available in fee-for-service medicine. The statistical limits of applying quality assurance measures based on large samples to patients with disabilities are presented.

Quality in health care also depends on the continued existence of academic medical centers, wherein subspecialists deal with complex medical problems. Through the creation of new knowledge and exposing trainees or residents to the most difficult cases, often at less than their true costs, these programs are expensive and easy targets for cost containing efforts. Chapter 7 is concerned with the impact of managed care on the capacity of these "centers of excellence" to continuously rebuild the infrastructure of medicine.

Managed care provides an opportunity to work toward mutually desired goals with public health organizations such as state maternal and child health programs. Chapter 8 focuses on the extent to which these partnerships have been created, the structural features of managed care organizations, and the existent public health programs that embody a limited congruence of aims of these two entities, as well as what needs to be done in the future.

Consumer protection has been discussed in the halls of Congress for much of 1998. Chapter 9 provides a brief account of "bill-of-rights" legislation on the legislative agenda and how it came that the legislation was finally passed in the United States House of Representatives and stalled in the Senate. The law that almost made it through Congress in 1998 is reviewed to determine its strengths and weaknesses for consumers with disabilities.

Finally, in chapter 10 I discuss some of the unresolved issues regarding disability and managed care.

REFERENCES

Birenbaum, A. 1981. *Health Care and Society*. Montclair, NJ: Allanheld, Osmun.

Lagnado, L. 1998. "Personality change: Old-line Aetna adopts managed-care tactics and stirs a backlash." *Wall Street Journal* (July 29th): A1, A6.

Mills, C. W. 1959. *The Sociological Imagination*. New York: Oxford University Press.

Murphy, R. F. 1987. *The Body Silent*. New York: Henry Holt and Company.

National Organization on Disability. 1998. *Closing the Gap: 1998. Expanding the Participation of Americans with Disabilities*. Washington, DC: NOD.

Nolan, C. 1987. *Under the Eye of the Clock*. New York: St. Martin's Press.

Self, T. W. 1998. "One man's battle with the managed-care monster." *New York Times* (July 13th): A17.

1

Disability, American Society, and Health Care

The study of disability can be approached from a number of different perspectives. Since my concern in this book is with changes in the health care system that impact on people with disabilities, it is important to discuss the way "disability" is defined officially as a vehicle for validating access to the various service systems. The health care system is but one of several that are important to people with disabilities. Most of the entitlements to services that have been the result of federal legislation followed wars that left many men with physical and mental disabilities. Members of Congress have stressed that there is a national obligation to assist those who served their country and were injured in battle.

In the United States over the past century these systems of assistance have evolved slowly to improve independence, productivity, and the integration of people with disabilities into our society. This assistance includes income maintenance, health care, vocational rehabilitation, and education benefits. There is still a long way to go to reach the above-mentioned goals as far as many people with disabilities are concerned, and the health care system is but one area that needs improvement.

Before discussing the vast institutional transformations of health care and the consequences for people with disabilities, I prefer to start from a social interactionist perspective, with an individual possessing the social skills involved in just being a member of society. The acquisition of a disability makes that person different both to him- or herself, in terms of performance of tasks of daily life, and to others. Acquiring a disability, or becoming a "significant other" of someone with a disability, involves a new social identity. Adaptation to this new fact about oneself is complicated by its social consequences or stigmatizing impact, what amounts to having a spoiled identity. This fully competent social actor, or, if young, one who has the capacity to become one, then has to learn how to deal with a diminished social status and play what is obviously an unwanted role. The acquisition of a disability equals the acquisition of a stigma—the individual is seen by others, and is often seen by him- or herself, as being tarnished or spoiled.

Societal and cultural analysis does not require that one be the role player or actor under discussion. Erving Goffman's classic insights into stigma did not appear to be based on personal experience. There are some occasions when the theoretical and the personal mesh in a powerful statement. Anthropologist Robert Murphy (1987), who acquired a severe disability, viewed the linkage between physical difference and social stigma this way:

> Disablement is at one and the same time a condition of the body and an aspect of society identity—a process set in motion by somatic causes but given definition and meaning by society. It is permanently a social state. . . . The onset of quadriplegia, I discovered, had placed me in a new social dimension. (195)

This acquisition of stigma is also a form of downward social mobility. Here Murphy relies on his anthropologic background to explain why this is so. People who cannot fully do basic things for themselves and who are perceived as not able to do for others cannot take part in a fundamental ritual of social life in any society—the principles of reciprocity, as identified by the French anthropologist, Claude Levi-Strauss (1969), in his brilliant work on kinship 30 years ago.

The more conformist the culture of a society, the more people with disabilities are shunned, their families are embarrassed by their presence, and little effort is made to accommodate people with physical limitations. In contemporary Japan—one of the most modern and developed societies technologically—individuals with disabilities "are often discouraged from working, from marrying, from going to movie theaters or restaurants" (Kristof, 1996: 3). In comparison, countries like Sweden, Denmark, and even the United States appear willing to promote the civil rights of people with handicapping conditions, even when full acceptance by others may not take place.

At the same time, the culture of the United States has evolved toward increasing concern about how we appear to others. The explosion of movies, along with magazines and radio advertising during the period between the world wars, all appealed to a nation of newcomers who were anxious about fitting in to the new urban society.

There was also the possibility now to change what nature had provided the individual with. Plastic surgery was invented during World War I to soften the facial disfigurement of wounded soldiers. It did not take surgeons long to figure out that Asians might like to eliminate "double eyelids," or Jews and Italians might find nose bobs a definite advantage as the standards of beauty were based on Anglo-Saxon and northern European models (Haiken, 1997). Eliminating stigmatizing features meant that one could compete more confidently in the world of work or when seeking a mate.

The late Erving Goffman (1963) made the problem of stigma a problem of everyday existence for the bearer. He dealt with the following questions: (1) What does it mean to play a stigmatized role in society? and (2) Why do people who are considered imperfect continue to act competently?

ON PLAYING A DISCREPANT ROLE

The answers to these riddles begin with a basic assumption about human beings and social life—they can take the role of the other. Being a fully competent member of society includes having a recognition of the meaning of membership and competency. This reflexiveness takes the form of what a member must possess and who is allowed to participate in particular social situations. Alternatively, knowledge of what it means not to be a member is part of the general role of the member. These rules or constitutive norms of social life are acquired relatively early in life.

Violations of these norms of social identity are one of the major concerns in Goffman's (1963) classic work. Every transgression of these norms in the form of a discrediting discrepancy between an actor's *expected* and *actual* identity calls into question the validity of these rules because those who cannot sustain competency may still seek to do so. The everyday grounds for judging others and oneself are made problematic because actors are uncertain about the kinds of claims that may be made by both the discrepant and the conventional individuals.

These "primal scenes" of social life, as Goffman observed, are often filled with embarrassment, awkwardness, and confusion. Generated by gaps between the way things are anticipated and the way they turn out, these encounters between discrepant and conventional individuals need to be made routine in order to end uncertainty on many levels; the discrepant person needs to be defined in a permanent way to end the disruptions to organized social life. Once societally designated agents redefine the discrepant person as being outside the conventional social order, the everyday grounds for the judgment of social identities are confirmed, thereby restoring beliefs of all members of society in the cultural formulas they have learned to follow (Garfinkel, 1956).

Moreover, the removal of uncertainty allows the stigmatized person to continue his or her membership in the social order, albeit assigned to a radically different master status. Once an individual acquires a disvalued identity, later encounters in his or her life as a stigmatized person acquire a predictable quality (Schutz, 1962). This process of recognition and acceptance of stigma reveals how society is able to restore belief in the cultural formulas when it is threatened, and which we all must follow, by labeling as soiled someone who was previously regarded as an unsoiled member of society. The process of stigma conference as a ritualized event helps to control the intensity and scope of stigmatization so the now disvalued person can continue with other responsibilities. Ironically, the people who involuntarily become deviants are asked to continue to hold up their end of things, to continue to conform, despite derogation and disappointment.

Conventional members of society question the competence of a person who fails to deal with "reality" or who denies what everyone else "knows" are the disadvantages of being disabled. The middle road is regarded as the wisest course because it confirms the conventional ideas about disability that are widely accepted in the culture. As stated sardonically by Goffman (1963):

> The general formula is apparent. The stigmatized individual is asked to act so as to imply neither that his burden is heavy nor that bearing it has made him different from us; at the same time he must keep himself at that remove from us which ensures our painlessly being able to confirm this belief about him. Put differently, he is advised to reciprocate naturally with an acceptance of himself and us, an acceptance of him that we have not quite extended him in the first place. (122)

Not every person who bears a stigma is disabled. There are stigmas acquired because of one's past behavior, ethnic group membership, or simply appearance without physical hinderance. A person who is extremely unattractive might be able to perform all the activities of daily living but might still be shunned or avoided. Physical beauty or even celebrity status, on the other hand, does not compensate for extreme loss of functions related to self-care, as, perhaps, the actor Christopher Reeve might agree.

Novelist and literary critic Leonard Kriegal regards the presence of disability in much the same way that Murphy saw it as a master status, but also as a barrier to being validated as a person. In his autobiographical account, Kriegel (1969) presents the other as failing to recognize the self present in the person with a disability:

> What the cripple must face is being pigeonholed by the smug. Once his behavior is assumed from the fact that he is a cripple, it doesn't matter whether he is viewed as holy or damned. Either assumption is made at the expense of his individuality, his ability to say "I." He is expected to behave in such-and-such a way; he is expected to react in the following manner to the following stimulus. And since that which expects such behavior is that which provides the stimulus, his behavior is all too often Pavlovian. He reacts as he is expected to react because he does not really accept the idea that he can react in any other way. Once he accepts, however unconsciously, the image of self that his society presents him, then the guidelines for his behavior are clear-cut and consistent. (424)

Given the almost existential quality to the interactionist perspective, as presented in the discussion of discrepant roles, there is a need to provide some "back story," as the writers of film scripts would say. Both the social origins and the political and economic consequences of disability require discussion. The incidence of disability in any society is not a result of random events. Spinal cord injuries and head trauma are associated with advanced economies that rely heavily on automobiles for transportation. Effective methods of caring for low-birth-weight newborns in intensive care units has meant that more infants survive often with lifelong handicapping conditions. Thirty years ago, infants with low birth weights did not survive, and consequently, in the past decades pediatricians were not evaluating and treating these children. Contemporary medical observers have characterized these conditions as the "new morbidities."

Childhood disability has been studied largely from the perspective of the coping response of the family to stress. The British scholar, David Thomas (1978), perhaps has done the most systematic work in this area, although his contribution took place over two decades ago. Much of the initial assessment or appraisal of the situation for parents may be derived from deeply held cultural beliefs. Regardless of culture, when a child becomes disabled, or is recognized as such during the early years of life, families invoke common-sense understandings related to the causes of the disability, hold to different expectations concerning the child's survival, and make judgments as to what success, or lack of it, this child will have in school, work, and family life (Groce and Zola, 1993: 1049).

A family's culture supports the interpretations and problem-solving efforts brought about by the presence of a child with a disability; it also is the force behind the coping strategies adopted. McCubbin and his colleagues call this construct a *family schema*, defined "as a structure of fundamental convictions and values shaped and adopted by the family system over time, which creates the family's *unique character* and serves as an overriding shared informational framework against and through which family experiences are processed and evaluated" (1993: 1064). Following the family schema, families develop *paradigms* or guidance mechanisms that "serve as a family framework intended to create, guide, change, affirm, and legitimate family behaviors and patterns of functioning" (1993: 1065).

This research team (McCubbin et al., 1993) developed two models: (1) family schema or family worldview and (2) family paradigms, with their specific beliefs and expectations for Anglo-American, Native American Indian, and Native American Hawaiian cultures. In the family schema model, family values and convictions are identified, while in the family paradigm model, specific domains of family functioning are viewed as derived from the family schema. Disability, for example, is defined differently by the three ethnic groups analyzed. Briefly, Anglo-Americans view it as foreign or intrusive on the family; Indians conceive of it as part of a general pattern of harmony and disharmony; and Hawaiians see disability as part of wellness or normal. It follows that families from these three very different ethnic groups would vary as to the perceived need to find treatment for the condition.

We live in a culturally diverse world, yet McCubbin and his colleagues noted that they started with a clean slate because there was a "dearth of research linking cultural and ethnic factors to the ways in which families respond to and cope with childhood illnesses and disabilities" (1993: 1063). Recognizing this diversity, some federal funding agencies such as the Maternal and Child Health Bureau and the Administration on Developmental Disability have given grants to study the social consequences of childhood disability, taking into account value and attitude differences held by different ethnic groups.

In American society most families and individuals from the mainstream culture, when faced with problems related to discrepancies between what is expected and outcomes, attempt to do something about it. American culture includes a well-recognized "can do" attitude. Doing often involves attempts at improving functioning.

A practice called rehabilitation has been called into being to deal with disability, whether among neonates or elderly stroke victims. The presence of disability and recognition that there are medical, educational, and vocational mediations available, even when disabilities are lifelong conditions, have also spawned new industries and businesses involved in rehabilitation.

What is the focus of rehabilitation? To answer this question we need a definition of disability that deals with both its social and functional consequences for the individual. The awesome mountaineer who used a prosthesis to compensate for a leg amputation, and who in 1998 climbed to the summit of Mount Everest, may not appear to be physically limited. Yet his identity, despite his heroics, may make him socially different.

Sociologist Gary Albrecht defines *disability* as a concept "referring to limitations in an individual's activity and role performance that require adjustments in the regimens of daily life and preestablished social relationships" (1992: 17). These limitations in activity and role performance can be located on a continuum, or they can be characterized as serious or minor, resulting, in some instances, in not being able to learn as well as others (e.g., mental retardation) or interfering with one's capacity to engage in a particular occupation (e.g., quadriplegia).

The presence of social stigma associated with a disability often creates constraints on the individual regarding how to present oneself to others. With some disabilities there are opportunities to hide the differentness (e.g., hearing loss). Other disabilities are more difficult to mask (e.g., a person who uses a wheelchair). One must deal with others who are uncertain about how to act toward the person with the disability.

The interactionist approach influenced the social science conceptualization of rehabilitation services, particularly in the 1960s when many of us saw striking parallels between people with disabilities and oppressed minorities. A major conference, "Sociological Theory, Research and Rehabilitation," held in Carmel, California, in March 1965 brought together an interesting array of sociologists who had made distinctive theoretical and empirical contributions to their discipline. Through this grant-funded working meeting, by invitation, these esteemed sociologists were to assist the Vocational Rehabilitation Administration (VRA), a branch of what was then the U.S. Department of Health, Education and Welfare.

The VRA commissioner, Mary E. Switzer (1965), presented the reason for the conference in a language disability activists today might find both inappropriate and appropriate:

Certainly dependency, in all its aspects, is a field that should concern sociologists. . . . So today, in the midst of our mounting prosperity, in the midst of the psychological climate of an affluent society, we have this mounting burden—the social, economic, spiritual burden of large numbers of dependent people. If you analyze why a good many of them are in a state of dependency, you have to come to the conclusion that they are there in large measure because of generations of prejudice against the provision of proper opportunity for them. (vii–viii)

Still, some of the strongest conceptual work at the conference undercut the suggestion that rehabilitation would make people with disabilities less dependent. The distinguished medical sociologist Eliot Freidson (1965) describes the field of rehabilitation as a form of social control, rather than a way of freeing people from dependencies. The field is seen by design to encourage stigmatization and, to some extent, new but different dependencies. Most important, rehabilitation was a way of imposing order on a chaotic part of life. The person who experiences a stroke, a spinal cord injury, or amputation must learn to live with a different body and with a new identity as one who is different from the conventional members of society. The reconceptualization, or social transformation, of people from the conventional to the unconventional must be done on a societal level, particularly when we believe that something must be done to fix what might not be broken or what cannot be fixed. In the beginning of his essay, Freidson lists the functions of rehabilitation. Some of these functions may be known to the participants and others may be unknown or latent. As with any process of sorting and validating, for example, entry into elite colleges, it might be best not to make the latent functions manifest.

> The institutions of the field known as rehabilitation may be said to carry on four activities. First, they specify what personal attributes shall be called handicaps. Second, they seek to identify who conforms to their specifications. Third, they attempt to gain access to those whom they call handicapped. And fourth, they try to get those to whom they gain access to change their behavior so as to conform more closely to what the institutions believe are their potentialities. (71)

The emphasis on stigma management has been eclipsed by more direct concerns related to independence and productivity. The prevailing definitions of disability currently in operation focus on functional limitations, or alternatively, deficits in performing activities of daily living (ADL) or instrumental activities of daily living (IADL). ADL consists of an individual's ability

- to get around inside the home;
- to get in or out of bed or a chair;
- to independently bathe, dress, eat, and use the toilet without assistance.

The more complex tasks related to IADL involve going outside the home, keeping track of money and bills, preparing meals, doing light housework, taking prescription medicines in the right amount at the right time, and using the telephone. Any enumeration of this population according to these criteria starts with people 15 years of age and over since younger children cannot be rated on some of these clearly adult activities (e.g., paying bills).

Definitions are sometimes created to establish eligibility for legal protection against discrimination. One that has withstood the test of time for over a quarter-century is the definition of physical or mental impairment derived from the Federal Rehabilitation Act of 1973:

> (A) any physiological disorder or condition, cosmetic disfigurement or anatomical loss affecting one or more of the following body systems: neurological; musculoskeletal; special sense organs; respiratory, including speech organs; cardiovascular; reproductive; digestive; genito-urinary; hemic and lymphatic; skin; and endocrine; or (B) any mental or psychological disorder such as mental retardation, organic brain syndrome, emotional or mental illness, and specific learning disabilities.

Note that the stigma-generating quality of a physical or mental condition is encompassed in this definition, for example, cosmetic disfigurement. There is also a noncategorical quality to this definition since no specific physical impairments are listed in Part A. Finally, the statute applies only to conditions that affect a major life activity, although what constitutes those activities remains open to broad or narrow interpretation.

In 1990 this same definition became part of the federal statute known as the Americans with Disabilities Act. It is this law that has been broadly construed recently to cover individuals who carry a potentially debilitating disease, whether it is a danger to the individual or his or her offspring. A 1998 five-to-four decision ruled that a woman with asymptomatic HIV infection was protected under the Americans with Disabilities Act. A major life activity was interfered with in her case because the act of procreation was impacted upon by carrying the virus. When a Maine dentist refused to fill her cavity in his office and said he would do so in a hospital, Ms. Sidney Abbott's civil rights were violated, according to the Supreme Court's majority opinion (Greenhouse, 1998).

Alternatively, there are definitions of disability for children or adults that often rely on whether there is interference with performance of major full-time roles, rather than capacity to accomplish some specific functions of daily life. Children who cannot attend regular school classes would be considered disabled. Adults who are not retired, but who cannot work, would also be so categorized. The number of days missed from school or work because of the presence of a health problem or other physical condition helps to determine the degree of disability. A person with epilepsy and frequent seizures would be considered disabled if this condition limited his or her capacity to attend classes or hold onto employment.

For some individuals, the degree of neurologic impairment that accompanies incapacity to accomplish some specific functions of daily life means that these conditions are encountered early in life and remain a lifelong problem. These conditions have been bundled together for entitlement purposes in federal legislation under the rubric "developmental disabilities." Since the passage in 1970 of the Developmental Disabilities Services and Facilities Construction Act, Public Law 91-517, the term groups together a number of heterogeneous conditions including mental retardation, cerebral palsy, epilepsy, and other conditions with "similar underlying neurological impairment." Later legislation included autism, spina bifida, and severe learning disabilities in this general category.

In 1975, the categorical definition gave way to a functional one. A five-part classification system uses the concept "substantial functional limitations" in three or more areas of "major life activities." The application of the concept of developmental disabilities in order to provide remediation may begin early in life. Young children with serious developmental delays and/or conditions identified at birth are not considered disabled but are candidates for being so classified. They may need interdisciplinary (e.g., educational and medical) interventions, mainly to prevent further deterioration. For those age 5 and older, a developmental disability is a severe, chronic disability that:

- is attributable to a mental or physical impairment or combination of mental and physical impairments;
- is manifested before the person attains the age of 22;
- is likely to continue indefinitely;
- results in substantial functional limitation in three or more of the following areas of major life activity: self care, receptive and expressive language, learning, mobility, self-direction, capacity for independent living, and economic self-sufficiency; and
- reflects the person's need for a combination and sequence of special, interdisciplinary, or generic care, treatment, or other services which are of lifelong or extended duration and are individually planned and coordinated; except that such terms when applied to infants and young children mean individuals from birth to age 5, inclusive, who have substantial developmental delay or specific congenital or acquired conditions with a high probability of resulting in developmental disabilities if services are not provided. (S.1284, 1993)

A person with a disability who leaves an entitlement such as Supplemental Security Income is taking a risk that public health insurance in the form of Medicaid or Medicare eligibility might be withdrawn. Once in the work force, an individual who is able to earn a living may not receive health care benefits, or alternatively, employers may fail to extend these benefits to a person who might be a heavy user of health services. Consequently, the loss of health care benefits to people with disabilities may prevent them from seeking gainful employment.

Health policy and disability experts have long noted the difficult situation that a person with a disability is placed in when he or she contemplates returning to the world of work. This is particularly evident for individuals who require a major regimen of drugs, often paid for by Medicaid. To encourage a return to work—and support independence and productivity—the Clinton administration in 1999 proposed "expanding Medicaid and Medicare to allow people with disabilities to retain their health benefits when they return to work" (Pear, 1998b). This is an exciting break with past policies and I, among many others, am anxious to see if this new approach will induce more people with disabilities into the work force, particularly at a time when unemployment is at a relatively low rate.

RATES OF DISABILITY IN THE UNITED STATES

How many people in the United States are disabled? The U.S. Census Bureau (1998) regards the Survey of Income and Program Participation (SIPP) as the most important current source of periodic data on the number and characteristics of people with disabilities. Surveys have their limitations when dealing with a condition that has many different ways of looking at it.

Social stigma may be at work indirectly because some people with disabilities may hide their differentness from surveyors. Alternatively, since there may be some financial or other incentives for claiming disability when in actuality it does not exist, there may be more people reporting to be disabled than other methods or ways of determining disability might confirm.

The strength of the SIPP is that it samples from the entire population and everyone has a similar chance, or equal probability, of being in it. In this way it avoids some of the bias that might be found when volunteers are solicited or only one area of the country is polled. People in rural, urban, and suburban areas have an equal probability of being selected for the sample.

A surprisingly large number of Americans have disabilities, although these disabilities are not all of the same level of severity. At the end of 1994, 20.6 percent of the population, about 54 million people, had some level of disability; and 9.9 percent, or about 26 million Americans, had a severe disability. The likelihood of having a disability increases with age, ranging from 1.7 percent for those people less than 22 years of age to 53.5 percent for those age 80 and older.

Who gets counted as having a disability often depends of which questions in the SIPP are considered. Using the same data source for 1990 and 1991, Fujiura and Yamaki (1997) estimated that 42.7 million persons in the United States, or 17.2 percent of the population, have physical and/or mental disabilities that impair their functional status. People with developmental disabilities, as previously defined according to functional status and being over the age of three, and identified by Fujiura and Yamaki (1997), constitute slightly less than one percent of the entire population of the United States. The use of functional status as the criteria for designation of disability may exclude from being counted as disabled those who admit to some difficulties in performing some activities of daily living but who still perform them.

When we count people age 6 years and older, in 1994, 1.8 million used a wheelchair and an additional 5.2 million used a cane, crutches, or a walker and had used such an aid for six months or longer. Deficits in seeing and hearing were even more common, with 8.8 million having *difficulty* seeing and 10.1 million having difficulty hearing. More significantly, the number *unable* to see was 1.6 million, and 1 million were unable to hear. A sensory deficit such as hearing loss does not necessarily entail dependence or functional limitations.

Specific questions were asked about their reliance on the use of other people, either volunteers or paid, for help with ADL. With children over the age of six included, the SIPP surveyors found that 4.1 million needed the assistance of another person with one of more activities of daily living. Over half of this group consisted of individuals age 65 years or older.

IADL questions were addressed by researchers to people age 15 and over. They found 15.3 million individuals who were unable to perform one or more functional activities and 9 million needed the assistance of another person with instrumental activities of daily living. Of the 9 million needing assistance with an IADL, 4.9 million were age 65 and older.

Of the 26 million people with a severe disability, 1.5 million were less than 22 years old; 6.1 million were 22 to 44 years old; 3.5 million were 45 to 54 years old; 4.5 million were 55 to 64 years old; 6.8 million were 65 to 79 years old; and 3.6 million were 80 years old or over. The Medicare-eligible population, those over the age of 65 and individuals below that age who were deemed fully disabled, consisted of 10.4 million people with severe disability. Given the limited incomes of many retired people, and the high cost of the multiple medications they take, health maintenance organizations, with their extended benefits for prescription drugs, look better and better. It is no accident that this is the part of the population today most rapidly joining health maintenance organizations (HMOs). While those with severe disabilities, and/or serious chronic illnesses, are probably remaining outside of HMOs, there needs to be some recognition that individuals of that age group may acquire severe disabilities after joining, a situation that presents problems for the risk-averse HMOs.

The substantial number of disabled people between ages 22 and 44 is not disproportionate for that age group in the general population. Yet this is also the age group that has the least health insurance coverage in the United States. Most of the shortfall in health insurance for this segment of the population has to do with a combination of employment where coverage is not available or, when available, is too expensive for young workers receiving modest wages to help pay for their share of the premiums, as required by their employers. Some young people, because they are healthy, moreover, feel invulnerable.

Health insurance does matter for low-income adults. Individuals without coverage may avoid medical care, hoping that a serious problem, such as intrauterine bleeding, will correct itself. People in low-paid employment often have to choose between insurance or something else that is worthwhile such as transportation to work.

Health insurance largely remains unaffordable to many working people, even when the employer offers to pay 50 percent or more of the cost. Despite a booming economy and a law to help people retain coverage even if they lose or change jobs, the high premiums for health insurance have led to an increase in the number of uninsured in the United States. It now exceeds 41 million (Pear, 1998a). People without insurance consistently report less access to care, whether they are healthy or have disabilities.

While youth may afford some protection, and most people with disabilities acquire them rather late in life, there is no guarantee that we will live into our sixties free of worry and care concerning functional deficits and limits to our abilities to do things for ourselves. There are also lifelong conditions that limit independence and productivity, and that affect a substantial part of the population. These conditions traditionally are ongoing concerns to policy makers and legislators. This is particularly the case with conditions such as mental retardation.

Limitations in a major life activity, linked to mental retardation, impact on many families. The 1994–1995 Health Interview Survey (HIS) had a disability supplement. The surveyors found that 0.78 percent of the population living in either general households or in formal residential support programs were identified as adults with mental retardation. Approximately 1,250,000 individuals were so designated in the most recent HIS-Disability Supplement.

Many of the services required by this population are paid for by federal and state funds, falling under the Medicaid program. In some instances, these individuals live in long-term care facilities, designated intermediate care facilities, that focus on their secondary medical conditions and functional limitations. Still other people with mental retardation live with their families or in group homes and receive assistance through flexible services and innovative case management or care coordination from the Medicaid-funded Home- and Community-Based Services (HCBS). Increasingly, Medicaid occupies more and more of the states' annual budgets. Some states are now attempting to consolidate health and long-term care services under a single managed care organization. While there is some merit to the idea of integrated services, the movement in this direction is driven by states seeking to contain costs. These decisions impact on families confronted by long waiting lists for services for their members with mental retardation and the individuals with this disability who have been encouraged during the last decade to choose their services rather then have them imposed on them. In fact, Medicaid-eligible individuals in general, whether disabled or not, may actually have more choice of managed care plans than those who get their health care coverage through their place of employment. There may be something to be learned from these experiences.

As we rarely realize, the fate of people with disabilities is of great moment to all of us. Since we entered the new age of managed care, well before the new millennium, the need for information as consumers and decision makers has increased mathematically. What is currently happening to people with disabilities and managed care is a preview, a coming distraction. Take warning—there are ways of organizing services that make it easy, or difficult, to get on with your lives. What will happen to the nondisabled as they are given financial incentives or simply forced by lack of choice into health maintenance organizations? Finally, readers, take note, that all of us, even the likes of "superman," are only a spine-jarring tackle, a poorly planned aquatic dive, or an equestrian accident away from becoming vitally interested in the cost, utilization, and financing of services for people with disabilities.

Focusing on what happens to people with disabilities when they are in managed care plans is of strategic import to the nondisabled. Many Americans worry about how well their managed care plan will work if they have complex medical needs. As the director of the District of Columbia–based

Center on Disability and Health, Bob Griss, is fond of saying, people with disabilities serve as the litmus test for the quality of the American health care system.

LIVING WITH DISABILITY

People with disabilities do not want to see themselves, nor do they wish to be seen by others, as a medical model, one that stresses their differences, limitations, and the sometimes substantial demand for resources that they place on the health care system. If anything promotes the idea that a disability generates stigma-conferring behavior on the part of others, it is the idea that individuals with disabilities suffer from a chronic condition. This condition is described by the Robert Wood Johnson Foundation (RWJF) report on chronic care in America (1996) as involving

> the presence of a long-term disease or symptoms; included in this category are physiological and psychological impairments, developmental disabilities, impairments caused by injuries, and secondary conditions, which are conditions related to the main illness or impairment that further diminish a person's quality of life, threaten one's health, or increase vulnerability to further disability.

A disability, whether acquired early or late in life, is a lifelong condition, making it different from a long-term disease that has acute stages, sometimes remissions, and often opportunities for disease management through medication or other treatments (e.g., chemotherapy, radiation). Contrasting even more with disabilities are the ways in which some long-term diseases now can be battled through surgical repair and organ replacement (cardiac bypass surgery, laser treatment of cataracts, or kidney transplants).

People who go through those kinds of treatments and repairs are often regarded as heroic because of the pain they underwent or lucky in that they caught something in time or were able to "beat the odds." In that sense the survivor is accorded some honor, much in the way that a soldier gets recognition for having gone through a major war zone even without doing anything noteworthy. There are campaign ribbons for soldiers who make it through famous battles, and for the patients who survive thoracic surgery there is admission to the special club called *Mended Hearts*.

Handicapping conditions do not resonate the same way in American culture. A child born without arms because his or her mother took thalidomide during the pregnancy to prevent a natural abortion in the 1960s is not accorded much status. While it may not be the person's fault, the acquisition of a disability still consigns the status of victim on the person. Pity is often considered appropriate, honor rarely.

Moreover, a disability does not confer any special privileges in the way that a serious chronic illness might excuse one from work or familial obligations while recovery is taking place. A permanent impairment involves limitations in performing activities of daily living, whether simple such as feeding oneself unassisted, or more complex such as paying bills. The presence of impairments triggers all kinds of responses that have their own consequences for social relationships. Even at a bare minimum, others may not be sure how to assist a person with a disability—how much that person can do independently or be capable of choices—or if a physical disability represents some mental impairment as well.

Disability is often difficult to disguise while many serious chronic illnesses are not readily visible in face-to-face interaction. Even a person who is a caregiver or companion to a person with a disability shares a bit of the stigma generated by the condition, although it has diminished intensity. Care givers may resent not only the burden of having to deal with the significant other's disability but also being considered different by outsiders. This significant relationship is not always known by others (Birenbaum, 1970). When one is a parent of a child with a developmental disability, this fact is not always known to all at the work place, church, or another sibling's school.

The world of disability has its fateful moments and its points of deciding how to deal with some facts that could be hidden but also could be discovered subsequent to the effort to cover them up. In sum, the person with an obvious disability, for example, a wheelchair user, must become adept at managing situations, such as acknowledging sympathetic remarks, while the person with a nonvisible chronic condition, one that might be controlled through medication, for example, epilepsy, has to deal with managing information (Goffman, 1963).

Negotiating social life for either person, given his or her spoiled identity and that he or she is not quite what others expect, is full of special concerns. Communication and easy interaction are affected since the person with a disability does not know what kinds of claims are going to be made on him or her by others. For the person with a disability, every new contact may be an event full of dread since the other may not be willing or able to pick up cues as to how the disabled person wishes to be treated. Consequently, there may be new expectations created for the individual because of the resulting stigma. These newly applied expectations are often widely shared. A person with a disability might be expected, for example, not to seek to engage in ordinary competitions for jobs or mates. Some activities, if undertaken by a person with a disability, might be viewed as inappropriate, such as when a person who is blind goes to a baseball game or a movie. Considered less inappropriate behavior for the blind might be attending a concert, singing in a choir, or swimming. Any of these reasonable activities might stimulate a second look or even a comment from others that shows some admiration for that person's pluck.

The movement for disability rights picked up steam in the 1960s, modeled after the civil rights movement and fueled by veterans of the Vietnam War who returned with disabilities from their wounds (Shapiro, 1993). The movement often failed to respect the medical control and medical definitions of their problems. They sought services that were not always "medically necessary" but that the consumers found useful. The quality of life was at issue. Consumers with disabilities did not care so much whether these services were deemed medical, educational, or vocational, so long as they were paid for and they had access to them. Integrated services, funded from different streams, were a goal and still remain out of reach for most of the disabled.

Despite the heroic effort of disability activists, the recent National Organization on Disability poll conducted in 1998 revealed considerable gaps in employment rates. Only 29 percent of the 1,000 people with disabilities interviewed of working age (18–64) work full or part time, compared with 79 percent of people without disabilities. Most of those respondents with disabilities who were not working would prefer to work.

Conducted by the Louis Harris organization, the survey found both physical and attitudinal barriers in many areas of living that keep people with disabilities from full participation in American society. As might be expected, life satisfaction for people with disabilities was approximately half the rate found among those without disabilities.

Most interesting was the comparative infrequency in socializing with close friends, relatives, and neighbors, and in going out to restaurants. There might be some social isolation that is due to unwillingness to be exposed to awkward, stigma-generating situations. Perhaps the lack of transportation is a factor at work here. Adults with disabilities identified inadequate transportation as a problem in their lives 30 percent of the time while adults without disabilities only saw this as a problem 17 percent of the time (National Organization on Disability, 1998).

Health care access was not one of the major issues raised by the 1998 survey. Yet transportation may be made more problematic for the disabled who join managed care plans with providers that are scattered widely about in a metropolitan region. The spread of managed care presents a new problem but also an opportunity to gain more care coordination than in the past.

NEW ORGANIZATION, NEW FINANCING, OLD PROBLEMS

There is widespread agreement that managed care may make things worse for people with disabilities, although the potential is there for creating seamless integrated service systems for this segment of the population. Recent nationally collected data on the growth of managed care and the experiences of people seeking health care suggest that some insecurities have been increased for people with disabilities.

The conversion of health insurance from indemnity coverage to managed care has forced both health care providers and consumer advocates to look closely at the consequences of this significant change for people with disabilities. As reported in *Health Affairs*, an authoritative policy journal, a recent survey of over 2,000 employers found that nearly three-quarters of U.S. workers and their covered dependents now receive coverage either through health maintenance organizations (HMO), preferred provider organizations (PPO), or the rapidly growing point-of-service plans, a type of coverage that provides limited insurance for going outside a health plan (Jensen, et al., 1997). Not to be outdone, the Health Care Finance Administration (HCFA) boasts on its home page on the Internet that it is the largest payer for managed care services in the United States, with 18 million Medicaid- and Medicare-eligible individuals now covered by managed care plans.

The greater efficiency in health care delivery introduced by HMOs has not done much to extend coverage to the uninsured, make health care more accessible than in the past, or eliminate financial woes for some consumers. Conducted by the National Opinion Research Center, a 1995 national telephone survey of 3,993 randomly selected respondents found 31 percent had experienced in the past year one of three core problems associated with the publicly recognized health care crisis of only a few years ago: an episode of being uninsured; a time when they did not get medical care that they thought they needed; or a problem in paying medical bills. Of course, there were those who experienced all three problems. Most important, people in fair or poor health, people with serious chronic illnesses, and people with disabilities were disproportionately over-represented in all three problem areas (Davis, Schoen, and Sandman, 1996).

In chapter 2, I will examine in more detail the discrepancies in utilization of health care services by people with disabilities when compared to groups of similar age or covered by the same insurance plan. I will also consider the special needs of individuals with two or more conditions, known in health care as *comorbidities*.

REFERENCES

Albrecht, G. 1992. *The Disability Business: Rehabilitation in America*. Newberry Park, CA: Sage.

Birenbaum, A. 1970. "On managing a courtesy stigma." *Journal of Health and Social Behavior* 11 (September): 196–206.

Davis, K., Schoen, C., and Sandman, D. R. 1996. "The culture of managed care: Implications for patients." *Bulletin of the New York Academy of Medicine* (Summer): 173–183.

Freidson, E. 1965. "Disability as social deviance." In M. B. Sussman, editor, *Sociology and Rehabilitation*. Washington, DC: American Sociological Association.

Fujiura, G. T., and Yamaki, K. 1997. "Analysis of ethnic variations in developmental disability prevalence and household economic status." *Mental Retardation* 35 (August): 286–294.

Garfinkel, H. 1956. "Conditions of successful degradation ceremonies." *American Journal of Sociology* 61: 420–424.

Goffman, E. 1963. *Stigma: Notes on the Management of Spoiled Identities*. Englewood Cliffs, NJ: Prentice-Hall.

Greenhouse, L. 1998. "Justices, 6–3, bar veto of line items in bills; see H.I.V. as disability. Ruling on bias law." *New York Times* (June 26th): A1, A18.

Groce, N. E. and Zola, I. K. 1993. "Multiculturalism, chronic illness and disability." *Pediatrics* 91 (May)(supplement): 1048–1055.

Haiken, E. 1997. *Venus Envy: A History of Cosmetic Surgery*. Baltimore, MD: Johns Hopkins University Press.

Jensen, G. A., Morrisey, M. A., Gaffney, S., and Liston, D. K. 1997. "Trends: The new dominance of managed care: Insurance trends in the 1990s." *Health Affairs* 16 (1) (January): 125–136.

Kriegel, L. 1969. "Uncle Tom and Tiny Tim: Some reflections on the cripple as Negro." *The American Scholar* 38: 412–40.

Kristof, N. D. 1996. "Outcast status worsens pain of Japan's disabled." *New York Times* (April 7th): 3.

Levi-Strauss, C. 1969. *Elementary Structures of Kinship*. Boston: Beacon Press.

McCubbin, H. I., Thompson, E. A., Thompson, A. I., McCubbin, M. A., and Kaston, A. J. 1993. "Culture, ethnicity, and the family: Critical factors in childhood chronic illness and disabilities." *Pediatrics* 91 (May) (supplement): 1063–1070.

Murphy, R. F. 1987. *The Body Silent*. New York: Henry Holt and Company.

National Organization on Disability. 1998. N.O.D./Harris Survey of Americans with Disabilities. Unpublished report. Washington, DC: National Organization on Disability.

Pear, R. 1998a. "Government lags in steps to widen health coverage." *New York Times* (August 9th): 1, 22.

Pear, R. 1998b. "Clinton proposes aid for disabled returning to jobs." *New York Times* (November 30th): 1.

Robert Wood Johnson Foundation (RWJF). 1996. *Chronic Care in America: A 21st Century Challenge*. Princeton, NJ: Robert Wood Johnson Foundation.

Schoen, C., Lyons, B., Rowland, D., Davis, K., and Puleo, E. 1997. "Insurance matters for low-income adults: Results from a five state survey." *Health Affairs* 16 (September/October): 163–171.

Schutz, A. 1962. *Collected Papers, The Problem of Social Reality* (Volume 1). The Hague: Martinus Nijhoff.

Shapiro, J. P. 1993. *No Pity: People with Disabilities Forging a New Civil Rights Movement*. New York: Times Books.

Switzer, M. E. 1965. "Remarks." In M. B. Sussman, editor, *Sociology and Rehabilitation*. Washington, DC: American Sociological Association.

Thomas, D. 1978. *The Social Psychology of Childhood Disability*. New York: Schocken.

2

Medical Care Financing and Utilization for People with Disabilities

For whatever reason, including disease management, pain management, or even acute depression, people with chronic conditions disproportionately use health services as compared to the general population (Robert Wood Johnson Foundation, 1996). They make more visits to the doctor, get hospitalized more, and use long-term care services more frequently than people without these conditions. Health economists estimate that this group accounts for most of the costs of health care in the United States (Hoffman, Rice, and Sung, 1996). The specialized health services required by people with disabilities may be more expensive than primary care because they involve intensive education and training and unique buildings and equipment that may not operate at full capacity all the time. Furthermore, patients may need to be monitored either as outpatients or inpatients for long time periods in order to determine how they can best respond to various kinds of therapies and prostheses and other appliances.

Consider what happens when a person needs to be assisted by a wheelchair. There are some surprises in store if the wheelchair-assisted person does not pay close attention to the way sitting can produce some scary moments. The need for medical care, particularly to deal with secondary conditions, is evident in Robert Murphy's autobiographical description of how medically and surgically involved his life became following the acquisition of pressure sores from sitting in a wheelchair. While the wheelchair is a source of mobility to those who cannot walk, it is also often the origin of decubitus ulcers, the result of skin breakdown when the person cannot move from one position to another for long periods of time.

This threat to health is particularly acute for quadriplegics who sit or lie in one position too long. As Murphy (1987) states:

> The constant pressure on one spot—usually one that is right over a bony prominence—prevents capillary circulation (already bad in quadriplegics) in the area, causing cells to die. The result is a small sore—no more than the size of a pinhead—which can expand into an ugly, gaping ulcer if the pressure is allowed to continue. (179)

People in wheelchairs are susceptible to this kind of serious skin breakdown, and if they have the arm strength, they are advised to lift their buttocks every 20 minutes to prevent decubiti from developing. There are also some cushions that help to prevent them from appearing. Ignoring these tiny red dots is perilous because the ulcer can grow both in depth and width, producing an infection that requires major treatment, including emergency plastic surgery to make repairs. In Murphy's account, failure to go to the doctor produced months of suffering, complex medical treatment, and the disruption of his professorial duties at Columbia University.

With managed care creating easy access to primary care providers and stressing prevention of disease, it seems plausible to suggest that wheelchair users or other people prone to skin breakdown would be able to get the care they need. This kind of access should reduce expensive hospitalization and the major involvement of infectious disease experts, plastic surgeons, and orthopedic surgeons, who all had to use their skills to restore Professor Murphy's capacity to sit, teach, and write, along with some of the more basic activities of daily living.

It is possible to prevent skin breakdown through the use of various kinds of seating and mattresses that reduce pressure. This kind of durable medical equipment, as this general category is called in the world of health insurance, is not always paid for by an HMO. Managed care plans and even state Medicaid will sometimes only pay for one brand of equipment, usually because it is less expensive than alternatives. By avoiding some expenses for durable medical equipment, payers do not recognize the substantial cost offsets that are involved. A person who avoids treatment for infected decubiti through the use of better, albeit more expensive, equipment will not need the various expensive medical and hospital services that Professor Murphy required to treat him. Secondary prevention works with disability and makes sense when a plan has a complete understanding of the needs of people with lifelong conditions.

Fast-forward from the experiences of Professor Murphy to 1998 and to Community Medical Alliance (CMA), the Boston-based HMO run by Bob Master. Utilizing nurse practitioners to visit quadriplegics at home to monitor for secondary conditions and make diagnoses and order treatments, this program shows how good managed care can be. In a striking opening to a major cover story on HMOs in *U.S. News and World Report* (1998), Joseph P. Shapiro, the author of *No Pity*, describes how Kerry Millett, under the care of Nurse Practitioner Mary Glover, is able to maintain the quality of his life and avoid hospitalization, thereby saving Medicaid, the payer for the services delivered through CMA, thousands of dollars annually. The article also cites instances where enrollees left the program and came back to it because they could not find this highly specialized form of primary care in other health plans. The following passage suggests why former enrollees come back and why most never leave CMA:

> Millett has been with CMA since it started in 1990 and has never had a bedsore or pneumonia. He credits Glover's quick response and CMA's emphasis on prevention. CMA will pay $16 to $30 a month for a special air mattress to prevent bedsores, which are common among quadriplegics because they often lie in the same spot for long periods of time. (68)

Spending for home health care, durable medical equipment, primary care, and mental health services keeps individuals with disabilities functioning and makes them less subject to secondary disabilities. In fact, the National Institute on Disability Rehabilitation Research (NIDRR), a branch of the U.S. Department of Education, has, in its recent proposed long-range plan, emphasized the interface between the individual and the environment as being a critical area for inquiry when looking at the adaptation process throughout the life span. When seen in this context, the health needs of people with disabilities take on new dimensions.

> The aging of the disabled population in conjunction with quality of life issues dictates a particular focus on prevention and alleviation of secondary disabilities and co-existing conditions and on health maintenance over the lifespan. (NIDRR, 1998: 57193)

With a critical number of Americans now living with various kinds of disabling conditions, federal legislation has accorded this part of the population a special status, entitling them to an enhanced learning environment through the Individuals with Disabilities Education Act, the successor to what was formerly known as the Education of All Handicapped Children's Act (1975); opportunities, starting in the 1950s, to receive subsidized vocational rehabilitation; and various antidiscrimination legislation, culminating in regulation of private enterprise as well as publicly funded organizations, as spelled out in the 1990 Americans with Disabilities Act.

This complex array of legislation was a result of actions taken and congressional lobbying by voluntary associations advocating for people with disabilities, including some self-advocate associations. The goals of productivity, inclusion, integration, and independence provided the backdrop for these substantial efforts to achieve as level a playing field as possible for Americans with disabilities.

The extension of life expectancy in the twentieth century started with improvements in access to food supplies, better sanitation, and improvements in the quality of the water supply. The development of emergency services has also extended life through rescue of those near death and the application of interventions for them. The capacity to prevent and treat viral infections, such as pneumonia, has also extended the lives of many people with serious disabilities. These people would have died in the past; now they live, often with serious disabilities. Not only are there more people alive through heroic intervention, but there are older Americans who, by virtue of access to medications that make it possible to survive with such conditions as congestive heart failure, have lived into their eighties and beyond. As Jerry Seinfeld might say, "not that there's anything wrong with that." While there is much that older Americans contribute to us, the problem for society is that they often cannot perform the ADL or IADL tasks.

The result has been the development of industries to assist these individuals in living in the community or nursing facilities. A substantial number of people with disabilities rely on equipment and supplies to not only keep them alive but also to improve the quality of their lives. To some extent they also need assistance from home care workers to maintain whatever functional performance exists and to help when they cannot fully take care of themselves.

The expenditures on these items make them likely targets for those who operate the new systems of health care where services are provided at fixed costs and risks are shared by providers with insurance companies. Managed care organizations, seeking to contain costs, often question whether the services and products generated by the rehabilitation industries are worth the expense, particularly since many of their enrollees will not regain functioning. Moreover, the home-based or nursing facility–based interventions constitute long-term care, for which, by contract, they are not responsible.

Similarly, medical management of disability has traditionally been in the hands of specialists while managed care organizations are built around the widespread use of primary care providers.

There is some survey evidence collected by the Houston-based Independent Living Research Utilization (ILRU) Program at the Texas Institute for Rehabilitation and Research (TIRR) that limited health insurance coverage, lack of access to health care providers, and exclusions based on pre-existing conditions mean that people with disabilities are not receiving the kind of care they need to maintain their optimal health.

The ILRU in 1994 compiled the results of a 12-page, 49-item self-administered survey from 750 people with disabilities. All of the respondents were volunteers and there was no probability sampling involved in finding the sample. Therefore, this survey sample does not represent all the people with disabilities in the nation or even in Texas. It does point, however, to some of the ways access to quality health care is important for people so they can get on with their lives. What follows are some of the highlights of this survey:

- Over one-third were unable to change jobs for fear of losing coverage because they had a pre-existing condition that would not be covered by the next employer.
- Almost one-half had to go without some needed items in order to pay for health care services.
- Almost one-half cited inadequate insurance coverage, given their medical needs.
- Three out of four said the high cost of treatment was a problem.
- Almost half said that physicians and other health care professionals lacked understanding of the health care needs and concerns of people with disabilities.
- Almost 80 percent needed services for disability-related health problems, and almost 70 percent said they need general health maintenance services.

The Houston-based Center for Research on Women with Disabilities more recently noted that people with disabilities reported delays in Managed Care Organizations (MCOs) in getting test results, being referred to specialists, scheduling procedures, and getting prescriptions filled (Chrzanowski, 1998). Anecdotal evidence suggests that there are many problems to work out. Late reporting of test results means, for example, that a person with post-polio syndrome with a urinary tract infection will not get treated in a timely manner. Lack of access to a urologist with experience in treating people with spinal cord injuries meant that another person had to wait six months to have kidney stones removed. Finally, a woman underwent potential loss of disability benefits when the tests did not confirm a diagnosis of lupus, a debilitating disease for which she was being treated.

The disabled, or in the modern language of choice, people with disabilities, have been fighting back for about 50 years, often against more formidable opposition than managed care organizations. A self-determination movement came out of the polio epidemic in the United States in the late 1940s. The youngsters who were subject to this disease refused to remain in institutions and back wards. They were not afraid to show themselves in public and demanded that service systems and their providers listen and then create support systems.

DISABILITY AND UTILIZATION OF HEALTH CARE SERVICES

The population of the United States for analytic purposes can be divided into those with disabilities and those without. The data from the National Health Interview Survey of 1989 were analyzed by LaPlante, Rice, and Wenger (1995) to determine if people with a limitation in activity due to chronic illness or impairment, a way of defining disability, are more likely to see physicians than those not limited in activity. They also wanted to determine if insurance coverage increased physician contacts. Disability and/or the lack of insurance coverage are powerful predictors of physician use.

> Adults who are unable to perform their major activity (paid work or keeping house) contact their physicians almost 20 times a year. By contrast people who are not limited in their major activity have 3.9 contacts a year. Lack of insurance coverage also affects physician contacts. Uninsured adults unable to perform their major activity have 25 percent fewer physician contacts than those with insurance—15.6 versus 20.9 contacts. Among adults not limited in activity, physician contacts are 47 percent fewer for those without insurance than for those with insurance—2.3 versus 4.3 contacts. (Laplante, Rice, and Wenger, 1995: 1)

Similar results were found when hospital stays were compared among those with and without limits in activities and for those with and without health insurance. Note that these findings were compiled before managed care enrolled many Americans. While it is likely that lack of insurance will produce the same lower utilization rates today as it did in 1989, it would be interesting to see whether individuals with limitations in activities who are in managed care plans have as many physician contacts as in the past or as many hospital stays.

Restrictions in activity are often associated with two or more disabling conditions. In a subsequent analysis of 1992 National Health Interview Survey (NHIS) data, Trupin and Rice (1995) found that "People with multiple disabling conditions have poorer health and use more medical services than those with only one condition"(1). Furthermore, the average number of bed-disability days more than doubles for those reporting two or more conditions as compared to those individuals reporting only one condition.

Medicaid and Medicare, two publicly funded programs, cover half of all medical expenditures for people with disabilities. Trupin, Rice, and Max (1995), using data from the 1989 NHIS, found that "Public programs account for 37 percent of medical expenditures for adults aged 18 to 64 with disabilities, as compared to 11 percent for those without"(3). While out-of-pocket expenditures account for a lower proportion of all medical expenditures for people with disabilities than for those without, the former spend out-of-pocket more than twice the dollar amounts that those without disabilities do. This is especially noteworthy since those with limitations in activities are more likely to be at lower income levels than those without limitations in activities (McNeil, 1997).

The previous discussion notes that people with disabilities are heavy users of medical services and they often demand access to care when it is denied. It is not surprising that these efforts were supported by corporations that produced durable medical equipment and supplies that assisted individuals with disabilities to perform various functions of daily living. Moreover, providers of special educational services, vocational rehabilitation and training, personal assistance, independent living centers, group homes, and health care tailored to people with disabilities also found it important to find and sustain financial support for their activities. While independence and productivity might be goals for each individual, these producers and providers had to be guaranteed a market for their products, services, and interventions in order for these organizations and individual practitioners to perpetuate themselves.

AGE-RELATED DIFFERENCES IN UTILIZATION

Studies of children with disabilities and/or those with chronic conditions that require more attention than children in general are good sources of information about the disproportionate need for health services of the first two groups. A recent epidemiologic profile of children with special health care needs (CSHCN) used a new definition of this population to analyze the data available from the special 1994 National Health Interview

Survey on Disability (NHIS). This definition included children with chronic physical, developmental, behavioral, and emotional conditions as well as those who used health or related services to an extent beyond that ordinarily used by children (Newacheck et al., 1998).

The researchers analyzed the 1994 NHIS interviews with parents of over 30,000 children under the age of 18. When compared with all children combined and children without special health needs, the CSHCN sample had a significantly higher use of health services, as measured by the number of physician contacts annually, percent hospitalized, and the average annual hospital days per 1,000 children. This population not only used health services more than the comparison groups but was also more likely to have bed days due to illness and higher rates of school absence due to illness, as can be seen in Table 1.

It is interesting, as an artifact of the chronicity of disability and the fact that these conditions are not life threatening, that the prevalence of conditions was higher among older children than younger children in the survey. Disability increases with age among children, as it does dramatically at the other end of the age range. Contributing to this age-related difference among children is the fact that many conditions are not detected until later years, particularly developmental, behavioral, and emotional conditions. It may not be until the child enters school that some of these differences be-

Table 1
Utilization of Health Services and Health Status for Children with Special Health Care Needs in the United States in 1994

	All Children	CSHCN	Children without Special Health Care Needs
Health Status			
Average Annual Bed Days due to Illness	2.8	6.1	2.0
Average Annual School Absences Due to Illness	3.6	7.4	2.0
Use of Health Services			
Average Annual Physician Contacts	3.3	6.4	2.6
Percent Hospitalized in Past Year	3.1	7.4	2.2
Average Annual Hospital Days per 100 Children	225.0	691.0	122.0

come apparent to parents and teachers. Children with chronic conditions who have frequent absences from school or have many bed days may also be prevented from experiencing a quality of life similar to that of children who are more active, even when they might be identified as having the same conditions.

There is increasing attention being paid by federal agencies to the numbers of children with special health care needs, whether they are insured, and what kinds of care they receive. Some studies in the early 1980s established that children with chronic conditions but without health insurance were not getting access to health services as frequently as children with insurance, even when they had the same levels of severity (Butler et al., 1987). In 1985–1986, I was the project manager of the Maternal and Child Health Bureau–funded special project of regional and national significance looking into the cost, utilization, and financing of health care for children with severe developmental disabilities (Birenbaum, Guyot, and Cohen, 1990). The use of large data sets such as the National Health Interview Survey did not give us an accurate picture of these particular developmental disabilities. Surveys, based on probability samples of households of the United States, did not collect a sufficient number of cases for low-prevalence conditions. Therefore, it was difficult to determine with statistical rigor if there were variables that could predict utilization, whether it was having insurance or any other outcome of interest. Our team collected data through telephone interviews at 11 sites for 308 children and young adults under the age of 25 with autism and from 326 children with severe or profound mental retardation. These findings, regarding annual physician visits and hospital discharges, were compared to national data from the 1980 National Medical Care Utilization and Expenditure Study, the 1986 National Health Interview Survey, and the 1987 National Medical Expenditure Survey.

An individual's annual number of physician visits is defined as the sum of all visits to physicians' offices, hospital outpatient departments, and emergency rooms. Children and young adults with autism visit physicians about four times per year, about the same as the national average of 3.6 visits for those from birth through age 24. By contrast, children and young adults with severe retardation average about nine visits per year.

Two-thirds of the children with severe retardation had physical impairments that accounted for their high visit levels. Note that preschool children were going to hospital clinics, where specialists are available, at about five times the average rate, but were only going to physicians' offices at about twice the average rate. We found that the ability to walk half a mile separated low users of medical services from high users.

The annual number of short-term hospital stays is a standard measure of health care utilization. Not only does hospitalization indicate the presence of a serious medical condition in the child, but it also is the major health care expenditure on behalf of American children, despite its rare occurrence. The children in our study who lived at home were more frequent users of in-hospital care than the average child. Ten percent of the children with autism in the 5-to-17 age group were hospitalized during a year, compared to 3 percent of all children.

Another measure of hospital use is based on the frequency of hospital discharge per 1,000 people in the population. The discharge rate in 1986 for all American children, ages 5 to 17, was 38 per 1,000 children, but for children with autism it was about 100 per 1,000 children and for children with severe retardation about 400 per 1,000 children, due to the high incidence of comorbidity.

Finally, it should be noted that some characteristics that predict health care use in the population at large also hold true for these disabled children. The mother's educational attainment predicts higher use of preventive and habilitative care and lower use of emergency room services. Black children are less likely to receive medical attention than white children. Lack of insurance predicts lower health care usage.

A more recent analysis of 1992 Medicaid claims and eligibility files from four states (California, Georgia, Michigan, and Tennessee) for children with Medicaid billing of at least $10,000 confirmed that children with disabilities had much higher expenditure and utilization levels than Medicaid-eligible children who were not disabled. Disability was identified by whether the child was eligible for Supplemental Security Income (SSI), a program that provides case benefits and in most states automatic Medicaid enrollment. While the investigators found that expenditures for children with SSI were 2.9 to 9.4 times higher than for other children, when the 10 percent of children with high expenditures (i.e., at least $10,000 annually billed to Medicaid) were eliminated, the differences in expenditures narrowed greatly (Kuhlthau et al., 1998).

The literature on utilization of health services for adults shows similar results. A small proportion of the population accounts for most of the expenditures. In a cost-driven system, these patients are likely to be the targets of efforts to create greater coordination and to make sure that every service rendered is truly needed. Here is where the struggle over access to services begins, and as described and analyzed in chapter 5, it is a battle over contested terrain.

Conditions that impact on quality of life are very expensive—both in terms of costs for care and opportunity costs. Opportunity costs involve lost earnings or chances to improve one's earning capacity through school attendance. Arthritis, for example, is a major chronic condition that affects about 16% of the American population (Yelin and Callahan, 1996). It is the second most prevalent disability among American women today. It is difficult to disaggregate the costs of medical care for arthritis from other conditions that are categorized similarly. Still, the estimates are astounding. Not only are there direct medical expenditures of $72.3 billion annually to treat this condition and other related musculoskeletal conditions, including osteoporosis, but lost productivity is calculated at $77 billion.

It is no wonder that MCOs seek to turn cases of serious chronic illness, such as diabetes, over to disease-management teams that are organized to care only for specific chronic conditions. This concept of care requires a sufficient volume of cases to make it cost effective to deliver services in this manner. When these teams accept the patients, they also accept financial risk for the patients' care, making cost containment a part of the formula for recommending monitoring and the approval of therapeutic interventions.

Annual data collected by the Health Care Finance Administration (HCFA) makes it possible to compare all Medicaid enrollees with individuals designated as entitled to Medicaid because they are considered disabled. The Supplemental Security Income (SSI) and the Supplemental Security Disability Income (SSDI) programs' staff make these determinations for adults who cannot earn enough to support themselves and for children who show substantial evidence of being unable to be self-supporting later in life.

Data on this population make comparisons possible with others who are also Medicaid recipients. HCFA (1997) reports its data on utilization of services according to eligibility groups. Eligibility groups include the low-income aged, the low-income disabled, children in low-income families, and adults in low-income families.

In Table 2, all eligibility groups combined are compared with those designated as disabled for the year 1995 according to the usual types of health services paid for by Medicaid. The category disabled includes SSI-eligible children. A person receiving multiple services (e.g., inpatient hospital, physician, and outpatient services) is included once in the user count for each type of services and once in the total. By including the low-income aged in this comparison, the contrasts with the disabled are diminished. Nevertheless, there is a clear difference in utilization rates when the two aggregated groups and the persons with disabilities are compared. Furthermore, including the elderly particularly diminishes the contrast with regard to long-term care utilization (i.e., nursing facility use) and this category is not included in this comparison.

Table 2
**Percent Distribution of All Medicaid Persons Served by
Type of Service Compared with Medicaid-Enrolled Persons
with Disabilities for 1995**

	Inpatient Hospital	Physician	Outpatient Hospital	Home Health	Prescribed Drug
All Eligible	15.3	65.6	46.1	4.5	65.4
Disabled	20.9	74.6	56.5	12.6	78.0

For adults, similar findings obtain. Chevarley and Hendershot (1995) analyzed data from the 1993 NHIS and show that work disability affects one in eight adults 25 to 64 years of age in the United States. Because of low incomes, they are likely to have public insurance and a regular source of care, but are less likely to receive needed and timely care.

In a sample of 43,000 households containing about 110,000 people, all persons 18 years of age and older were asked questions about whether they have impairments or health problems that keep them from currently working at a job or business, or limits the amount of work they can do. If a work limitation is reported and is associated with a chronic health condition or impairment, the person is considered to have a work disability. Whether or not they had insurance or a regular source of care, many persons with work disability reported not getting needed care or delaying care due to the cost. Those with no health insurance and no regular source of care were most likely to report not getting needed care or delaying care for financial reasons.

People with disabilities need to be regarded as having the same needs as everyone else. This means that promotion of fitness and improvement in one's general outlook are matters for concern for both professionals and their clients or patients. Disability has enormous consequences for the quality of life of the person with chronic and other conditions. It has pervasive effects on the quality of life of millions of Americans. Yet, as noted earlier in the discussion of children and utilization of health services, missed days of school, and bed days, there are wide variations within the same category of chronic conditions in activity levels and restricted days.

Recently, rehabilitation specialists have begun to consider how health-promoting behaviors can impact on people with such debilitating conditions as multiple sclerosis (MS) (Stuifbergen, 1995). A preliminary analysis of a convenience sample of 61 individuals with MS found a positive relationship between health-promoting behaviors and the quality of life.

We often do not recognize that health promotion is important because of the comorbidities that exist alongside chronic conditions of all types. Another way to determine the extent of utilization of health services is to review records of people with disabilities to find out whether they have secondary chronic conditions. In my abstract and poster presentation (1995) of the evaluational study I co-directed (with Phillip Davidson) of the New York State Home- and Community-Based Waiver Program, I reported that, in a random sample of 200 individuals identified primarily as mentally retarded, 65 percent had a secondary disability. The most frequently found secondary diagnosis was epilepsy, followed by cerebral palsy, behavioral or psychological disorders, and autism. In an additional 24 percent of cases there was a third disability, with cerebral palsy the most frequent diagnosis. Finally, a fourth diagnosis was found in 8 percent of the cohort.

Access to quality medical care for adults with developmental disabilities is a major concern for agencies with policy responsibility for this population. In 1998, the National Institute on Disability and Rehabilitation Research set aging with mental retardation as one of its funding priorities for the fiscal year 1998–1999 because: (1) there is evidence that lifelong exposure to psychotropic and anti-seizure drugs has generated secondary conditions (osteoporosis or tardive dyskinesia); (2) treatment of normal diseases of aging (e.g., hypertension) pose problems for providers attempting to communicate about diet, exercise, or medication adherence with aging persons with mental retardation; and (3) the health status and needs of older women with mental retardation has received little research attention. With 80 percent of adults with mental retardation living at home, and with many known to the service system, there is an excellent opportunity available to ensure that access to health care is optimized (Department of Education, 1998).

Observers over the past decade have noted that people with disabilities, particularly those with developmental disabilities, are living longer. Consequently, there are all kinds of service requirements that have to be met for a population that is more likely than in the past to outlive care givers. Sociologist and public health expert Louis Rowitz (1989) was among the first scholars to recognize these demographic trends.

It is also noteworthy that observers of these trends have found that the effects of aging on people with disabilities have not been studied systematically. Anecdotal information collected by people with disabilities suggests that there may be general deterioration that is age related even when the condition is not considered a progressive disorder, such as multiple sclerosis or Parkinson's disease.

Consider the aging process for people with cerebral palsy. Seltzer and Luchterhand (1994) suggest that

> they will experience a decline in functional performance, physiological changes, pain, and restrictions in their daily social and emotional activities at an earlier age than their age peers without cerebral palsy. (120)

These changes are devastating for a person with cerebral palsy attempting to get around without the use of a wheelchair. There are multiple orthopedic problems that emerge in midlife that impact on the functioning involved in ordinary activities. In sum, the emergence of these problems calls into question the person's resolve to participate in social activities or continue to be employed.

PSYCHIATRIC DISORDERS

Perhaps no disabilities are more pervasive than those associated with emotional distress. These conditions, particularly depression and other mood disorders, are very widespread and have high rates or recurrence, relapse, and chronicity. Reporting in 1995, Judd concluded that approximately 11.3 percent of all adults are afflicted by depressive disorders during any one year, making this disease or disability one of the most common in modern society.

The condition of depression is "associated with significantly greater physical limitations, more dysfunction in ability to perform one's social and occupational role and with increased bed days and poor estimation of personal health"(5). Judd came to the realization that this is an important public health problem. It also should be noted that the social costs of mood disorders are high because of the heavy impact on significant others, who often must serve as care givers.

Anxiety disorders such as panic disorder, phobias, or obsessive-compulsive disorder are very common and often are associated with depression and other mood disorders. Data from the National Institute of Mental Health Epidemiological Catchment Area Program were analyzed by Leon, Portera, and Weissman (1995). They found over 6 percent of the men and 13 percent of the women in a sample of 18,571 had suffered from a clearly identifiable anxiety disorder in the past six months. Nearly 30 percent had turned to the health care system in that study period to receive help with either emotional or alcohol- or drug-related problems. Individuals with anxiety disorders were also more likely to seek specialized care from the mental health system than those with other conditions.

A more recent study of the medical and pharmacy claims for the period 1990–1994 for over 700,000 claims in the United States found that people with depressive illness consume two-to-four times more general medical resources than patients without mental illness (Croghan, Obenchain, and Crown, 1998). Utilization (and, of course, expenditures) for patients with one or more comorbid conditions, especially those related to anxiety, is much higher than for patients with depressive illness and no comorbid conditions. Early intervention may also produce major "up front" expenses but may produce better outcomes and reduce the need for, or the length of, hospitalization later in the acute course of the illness.

New approaches to care are of major concern in the field of mental health since payers are unwilling to sustain the rising cost of this kind of care. There is some evidence to suggest that disease management programs for mental health services are able to deliver the same quality of service at about 22 percent less cost. Massachusetts was the first state to introduce a statewide specialty mental health managed care plan for its Medicaid program. Reduced lengths of stay, discounted fees from therapists and hospitals, and fewer inpatient admissions accounted for most of the savings (Callahan et al., 1995). Some substitutions for inpatient care were introduced.

Nevertheless, some unwanted findings did result with regard to children and adolescents who received services. Readmission rates increased slightly, and providers for this group were more dissatisfied when working under managed care than before the new ways of delivering care were adopted. Despite these mixed results, the authors concluded that this experience supports the use of managed care for mental health and substance abuse services for a high-risk population.

The experiences recounted here are based on a diverse population with disabilities and with many different medical needs. Following a 1994 conference funded by the Health Care Financing Administration's Office of Research, a report on health care for persons with disabilities identified managed care as being both an opportunity and a threat to this population. The editors of the report captured—with a broad Chinese calligraphy brush—the kinds of issues that are raised about managed care for special needs populations (Wiener, Clauser, and Kennell, 1995):

> New initiatives for managed care offer the potential for better service to the disabled population as well as potentially significant cost savings. New approaches that combine both acute and long-term care could provide a seamless system that would meet the total needs of each individual. However, with their emphasis on reducing use of services, limiting the choice of providers and cutting back on use of specialists, managed care organizations

possibly threaten the provision of high-quality care to disabled persons. It is therefore critical to evaluate the impact of managed care. (13)

What is it about managed care that causes so much concern? Is this insecurity and sense of crisis temporary—a result of the social dislocation caused by the transformation of the organization and financing of health care to contain costs—or are there permanent features of managed care organizations to which people with disabilities need to be especially sensitive?

REFERENCES

Birenbaum, A. 1995. "The Home- and Community-Based Waiver Program in New York State: An analysis of services recommended and received." Published abstract and poster presentation. *Annual Abstracts of the Association of Health Services Research Annual Meetings*: 72.

Birenbaum, A. 1970. "On managing a courtesy stigma." *Journal of Health and Social Behavior* 11 (September): 196–206.

Birenbaum, A., Guyot, D., and Cohen, H. J. 1990. *Health Care Financing for Severe Developmental Disabilities*. AAMR Monograph 12. Washington, DC: American Association on Mental Retardation.

Butler, J. A., Singer, J. D., Palfrey, J. S., and Walker, D. K. 1987. "Health insurance coverage and physician use among children with disabilities: Findings from probability samples in five metropolitan areas." *Pediatrics* 79: 89–98.

Callahan, J. J., Shepard, D. S., Beinecke, R. H., Larson, M. J., and Cavanaugh, D. 1995. "Mental health/substance abuse treatment in managed care: The Massachusetts Medicaid experience." *Health Affairs* 14 (Fall): 173–184.

Chevarley, F. M., and Hendershot, G. 1995. "Access to health care among persons with disabilities: United States." In the *Proceedings of the 25th Public Health Conference on Records and Statistics*. Washington, DC: National Center for Health Statistics.

Chrzanowski, L. J. 1998. "Study reports MCOs pose barriers for disabled people." *Disability News Service's E-NEWS* (August): 3.

Croghan, T. W., Obenchain, R. L., and Crown, W. E. 1998. "What does treatment of depression really cost?" *Health Affairs* 17 (July/August): 198–208.

Department of Education, National Institute on Disability and Rehabilitation Research. 1998. "Notice of proposed funding priorities for fiscal years 1998–1999 for rehabilitation research and training centers." *Federal Register* (May 4th): 24717–24721.

Goffman, E. 1963. *Stigma: Notes on the Management of Spoiled Identities*. Englewood Cliffs, NJ: Prentice-Hall.

Health Care Financing Administration. 1997. Tables 76 and 77. *Health Care Financing Review: Medicare and Medicaid Statistical Supplement, 1997.*

Hoffman, C., Rice, D., and Sung, H. 1996. "Persons with chronic conditions: Their prevalence and costs." *Journal of the American Medical Association* 276: 1473–1479.

Judd, L. L. 1995. "Mood disorders in the general population represents an important and worldwide public health problem." *International Clinical Psychopharmacology* 10 (Supplement) 4 (December): 5–10.

Kuhlthau, K., Perrin, J. M., Ettner, S. L., McLaughlin, T. J., and Gortmaker, S. L. 1998. "High expenditure children with Supplemental Security Income." *Pediatrics* 102 (September): 610–615.

Laplante, M. P., Rice, D. P., and Wenger, B. L. 1995. "Medical care use, health insurance, and disability in the United States." *Disability Statistics Abstract* 8 (May).

Leon, A. C., Portera, L., and Weissman, M. M. 1995. "The social costs of anxiety disorders." *British Journal of Psychiatry Supplement* (April) 27: 19–22.

McNeil, J. M. 1998. "Americans with disabilities." *U.S. Census Bureau.* http://www.census.gov/hh...p/disab9495/asc9495html

McNeil, J. M. 1997. "Americans with disabilities: 1994–5—Table 8." *U.S. Census Bureau.* http://www.census.gov/hh...pp/disab9495/ds94t8.html

Murphy, R. 1987. *The Body Silent.* New York: Henry Holt and Company.

Newacheck, P. W., Strickland, B., Shonkoff, J. P., Perrin, J. M., McPherson, M., McManus, M., Lauver, C., Fox, H., and Arango, P. 1998. "An epidemiologic profile of children with special health care needs." *Pediatrics* 102 (July): 117–140.

NIDRR. 1998. "National Institute on Disability and Rehabilitation Research; Notice of proposed long-range plan for fiscal years 1999–2004." *Federal Register* (October 26th): 57190–57219.

Robert Wood Johnson Foundation (RWJF). 1996. *Chronic Care in America: A 21st Century Challenge.* Princeton, NJ: Robert Wood Johnson Foundation.

Rowitz, L. 1989. "Trends in mental retardation in the 1990s." *Mental Retardation* 26: 115–117.

Seltzer, G. B., and Luchterhand, C. 1994. In M. M. Seltzer, M. W. Krauss, and M. P. Janicki, editors. *Life Course Perspectives on Adulthood and Old Age.* Washington, DC: American Association on Mental Retardation.

Shapiro, J. P. 1998. "There when you need it." *U.S. News and World Report* (October 5th): 64–72.

Stuifbergen, A. K. 1995. "Health-promoting behaviors and quality of life among individuals with multiple sclerosis." *Scholarly Inquiry for Nursing Practice* 9: 31–50.

Trupin, L., and Rice, D. P. 1995. "Health status, medical care, and number of disabling conditions in the United States." *Disability Statistics Abstract* 9 (June).

Trupin, L., Rice, D. P., and Max, W. 1995. "Who pays for the medical care of people with disabilities?" *Disability Statistics Abstracts* 13 (November).

Wiener, J. M., Clauser, S. B., and Kennell, D. L. 1995. *Persons with Disabilities: Issues in Health Care Financing and Service Delivery*. Washington, DC: The Brookings Institution.

Yelin, E., and Callahan, L. 1996. "The economic cost and social psychological impact of musculoskeletal conditions." *Arthritis & Rheumatism* 38 (10): 1351–1362.

3

Full-Blown Managed Care

Managed care defies our common-sense understanding of value in the world of work and in the area of health care. Managed care advocates challenge conventional wisdom when they claim that doing less produces a greater outcome for the patient than taking action as well as promoting the common good. Economists in the nineteenth century believed that all work can produce something of value. Usually, the more we do, the better off we are. Thus, more value is added to what is produced. For example, when you extract iron ore from the ground, and add carbon to it under intense heat, steel is produced. For some economists, human labor is what creates the value in the product not just the fact that now it can be sold in the marketplace. A similar process takes place in protecting human life and fighting disease through medical interventions.

In health care, if you immunize a child, that child is protected from a disease, and the value is realized by the intervention. This is a decisive form of medical technology, sometimes referred to as a preventive intervention. Managed care is a unique form of health care delivery because it is premised on the idea that often, in medical care, less is more. What produces value in managed care is a good health outcome rather than medical intervention. Not every visit to a doctor is necessary; nor is every test conducted, medication prescribed, or placement in an intensive care unit going to produce an effective outcome. Ideally, medicine should be ruled by rationality and efficiency in the choice and implementation of evaluations and treatments. This means that the variability between providers not only should be, but can be, eliminated, and the only factors that should make a difference in deciding who to treat and what treatment to undertake are the nature of the patient's disease or injury.

Behind this kind of thinking is a very powerful guideline: we, as a country, or a planet, cannot treat everything and we need to make distinctions between treatments undertaken on the basis of effectiveness and those made because of cost. Managed care introduces explicit rationing, based on looking at an array of variables that can influence outcomes. Some treatments may be ruled out because of the patient's age or frail condition. Few surgeons would repair a hernia in a 99-year-old man. In some countries, for example, in the United Kingdom, where an effort is made to limit the resources given over to health care, this kind of rationing is formulated into rules that all providers, and patients as well, must live under. Usually, these restrictions are based on scientific evidence of the limited benefit of expensive treatments for certain sectors of the population. The rules may prevent older people from gaining access to the government-run dialysis units to treat end-state renal disease. If they want to pay out-of-pocket, and can afford it, they may find a private facility that can accommodate individuals with poor kidney functioning.

The complex and expensive American health care system—with 15 percent of the population uninsured—also rations, but it is on a covert, rather than an overt, basis. Those without insurance use services at lower rates than those covered by any kind of health plan. However, it does not follow that the young and the healthy are the uninsured. What the uninsured tend to share in common is an inability to afford insurance.

People without insurance consist of some healthy individuals as well as a substantial number of at-risk individuals who are underutilizers of regular sources of care. In turn, they may forgo a visit for some preventive intervention to avoid spending out-of-pocket. While not every woman who avoids a Pap smear is subject to cervical cancer, early detection among the few who test positively for that disease saves lives as well as more costly treatments in advanced stages of the disease.

One also has to look at the demographics to understand why we as a nation need to cover everyone in the population. Americans constitute an aging population, and this means that we will be subject to chronic conditions such as heart disease and cancer. An analysis of 1987 and 1990 national data found that over 45 percent of noninstitutionalized Americans have one or more chronic conditions. In the aggregate, the treatment of chronic diseases accounts for three-fourths of total health expenditures in the United States (Hoffman, Rice, and Sung, 1996). The majority of people with chronic conditions hold jobs and are not elderly. Little is known about how well managed care and health maintenance organizations provide care, not cures, for these disproportionate users of health care.

As far back as 1993, some skepticism was expressed by policy analysts Mark Schlesinger and David Mechanic about how well—under conditions of competition and fixed budgets—health maintenance organizations provide for people with serious chronic illnesses and disabilities. Moreover, the potential problems identified in managed care for insuring people with chronic illnesses led these policy analysts to suggest the development of various forms of reinsurance to protect health plans; a broader benefits package than most plans offer; and sophisticated case management models (Schlesinger and Mechanic, 1993: 136).

HEALTH MAINTENANCE ORGANIZATIONS

It has often been observed that the real consumers of health care services are physicians rather than patients. When doctors order up tests or hospitalize patients, they encounter no financial risk in traditional fee-for-service medicine; and third-party payment softens the economic blow to the patient who might question the absolute necessity of a procedure or a hospital stay. Under third-party payment, patients freely choose providers, and there is no advance agreement to serve a particular panel of patients. Integrating payment and provider in the same plan is a key innovation in American health care because it makes discipline over physicians possible.

A health maintenance organization (HMO) is both a financial plan and an organization of services for a specific population of subscribers. In this arrangement, a fiscal agent agrees to be accountable for all stipulated health services for the subscribers at a fixed price. This combination payer and provider assumes financial risk for those covered by the plan. Unlike straight indemnity insurance, HMOs exercise various kinds of controls over providers and members. Those who enroll in the plan do so voluntarily and pay this price regardless of whether or not they use the services available. An advantage for the covered is that they have no first-dollar or deductible obligations and generally pay only a modest co-payment when they see a doctor. In some HMO arrangements providers do not even collect the small co-payment because it generates so little in the way of revenue and incurs an overhead cost to handle. A major component of the economic arrangements of HMOs is that all major hospital costs are paid for out of the combined capitation fees. Hospitals agree to make beds available in advance to the HMO at a discounted price or the HMO owns hospitals. Either way, HMOs try to limit hospital utilization because it is a major proportion of the costs that will be taken from income.

HMOs contract with providers in various ways to get them to deliver services. In staff-model HMOs, such as Kaiser Permanente and Puget Sound, the physicians and other providers are salaried and work directly for the HMO, which also provides all nonmedical services. Doctors assume no financial risk in this model. Other arrangements use various financial incentives for either groups of physicians or solo practitioners to keep costs down.

The group-model HMO usually provides the hospitals and other physical facilities and employs the nonphysician clinical staff. It also provides the administrative support staff. The HMO contracts with one large (professionally autonomous) multiple-specialty medical group practice for physician services. The HMO pays the medical group a monthly amount per member to provide services (Freeborn and Pope, 1994: 21).

Within each group, physicians usually work only for that HMO, are salaried, but with monetary incentives and penalties are at some financial risk. These groups are made up generally of a very large number of physicians and provide a comprehensive set of medical services.

An expansion of the group model is the "network model," wherein an HMO contracts with several physician groups, but with the same capitation arrangements to cover members. Nonphysician services are provided by the group, which also assumes financial risk.

Finally, the fastest-growing model in the 1990s is one where individual physicians, forming an independent practice association (IPA), contract to care for covered individuals, usually on a heavily discounted fee-for-service basis. There is use of risk-capitation in some IPAs. In this model the physician often belongs to several HMOs at the same time. Located throughout a region, IPAs permit consumers to make choices from a larger number of primary care providers and specialists than are generally found in the other models. In addition, providers are not subject to an integrated health service system. Enrollment growth in 1994–1995 showed a 22 percent increase in networks and IPA-model HMOs, compared with an 8 percent increase in staff-and group-model HMOs (American Association of Health Plans, 1996: 2).

HMOs are said to have a competitive advantage over traditional fee-for-service and third-party coverage because the enrolled achieve financial security as far as their medical expenses are concerned. In addition, capitation charges are considered to be lower than in straight indemnification insurance policies, whether group or individual, because providers have no incentive to do unnecessary work. Primary care doctors or physician extenders (nurse practitioners or physician assistants) act as "gatekeepers" to specialty care. Physician extenders are much less expensive to employ than doctors and do excellent work in primary care, particularly in doing the routine but highly important tasks necessary to keep people well. A United States Office of Technology Assessment (1986) review of all studies comparing the work of nurse practitioners with physicians confirms this view.

Doctors who tend patients in managed care are driven by the concern to avoid unnecessary resource utilization. HMOs encourage patients to have regular examinations while not overusing expensive kinds of interventions. Managers of HMOs try to establish primary care as the front line of service and have an incentive to get providers to do preventive interventions and early detections through simple tests (e.g., the Pap smear) in order to avoid more complex interventions and hospitalization later on. Sometimes providers also are given financial incentives to follow this model of service rigorously.

Although HMOs have been around for 60 years in the United States, federal legislation that provided financial incentives to start up for-profit prepaid programs initiated a rapid and enormous expansion of members in the 1980s. The Tax Equity and Fiscal Responsibility Act of 1982 expanded the market by making it easier for Medicare and Medicaid beneficiaries to enroll in HMOs. Marketing was intense. I recall that in 1984 the Chicago radio air waves were full of advertisements for HMOs, aimed at the senior citizen set. Today HMOs increasingly serve a larger and larger proportion of the over-65 population, with HMOs reporting in 1996 the development of many new Medicare risk contracts or plans to do so. Similar trends for contracts were found with regard to the Medicaid-eligible population, with many new programs coming on line.

Finding resources to deliver managed care became less and less of a problem for HMOs as the market favored buyers rather than sellers of health services. The oversupply of hospital beds and physicians during the 1980s and 1990s created a strong impetus for providers to sign on with profit-making and nonprofit HMOs, guaranteeing a predictable and large volume of resources. Even august institutions found HMOs attractive. In response to losing patients, teaching hospitals with affiliations with prestigious medical schools began to create joint ventures with HMOs. In the last decade, insurance companies and state-organized Blue Cross programs began to sell HMO services to subscribers. In sum, a great transformation in the organization of providers came about with these new market considerations.

HMOs were believed to be economically viable because of their success in keeping people out of hospitals. In addition, the nonprofit HMOs essentially catered to young and healthy families who needed routine care but rarely had the need for hospitalization. Large employers led the way in encouraging their workers to join HMOs. The financial advantage to subscribers—no deductible and no serious co-payment for office visits—was a major selling point in getting conversions from traditional insurance coverage.

Growth in HMO membership has been phenomenal during this decade. Research centers and professional associations followed these trends keenly. In 1989, InterStudy, a Minneapolis-based research organization, reported that HMO membership was at 32 million. The *American Medical News* (1991: 33), a publication of the American Medical Association, noted that an American Association of Health Plans study found that HMOs appear to be most successful in the nation's largest cities and those areas where they have been available the longest. The cities of San Francisco (46 percent) and Minneapolis-St.Paul (44 percent) led the way with the highest numbers of HMO members among all residents.

For employers, however, some of the HMOs' great economic appeal appears to be wearing out. Even if the enrollee gives them high marks, the corporations have found that annual increases in costs can approximate those of traditional indemnification plans or even those with managed care provisions. In some cases, businesses have dropped one or more of the several HMO plans available to their employees and dependents. However, with 545 HMOs operating nationally, as reported by the Group Health Association of America (GHAA) in 1993, there seemed to be no difficulty shopping for substitute plans. Moreover, reflecting both growth and diversity, this trade association has merged with the American Managed Care and Review Association to form the American Association of Health Plans (AAHP). By late 1996 the AAHP had more than 1,000 member health plans, providing coverage for over 100 million Americans nationwide.

Where did this concept come from? Is this just another foreign import, another Volkswagen or Honda? No, HMOs are truly an American product. One of America's major industrial magnates, Edgar Kaiser, will probably earn a place in American social history for his contribution to the extension of affordable health care to millions on the West Coast. In fact, Kaiser himself suggested that he was most proud of starting the Kaiser Permanente Health Care Partnership (Keene, 1971).

This partnership came from the modest need to provide modern health care in locations where such services were minimal. The urban development and agribusinesses of southern California were dependent on getting water from remote mountain areas, far distant from the coastal locations where cities were being built. Teams of construction workers were employed in the 1930s to build reservoirs and pumping stations, and to lay pipe for the aqueducts that carry water to the coastal areas and valleys. Sidney Garfield, a young physician, had tried to establish a private practice in towns near this construction. He found plenty of demand for his services among the construction crews but no way to receive adequate compensation. As a result, Garfield developed a scheme whereby each worker would contribute a small amount every week on a contract basis, paying in advance for any medical care he provided. In exchange for these payments, he agreed to provide all medical care, no matter how often required. Garfield even built a small mobile field hospital that could be moved on skids to follow the crews as the project advanced (Cutting, 1971: 17–18).

In 1937, some five years after Dr. Garfield started this program, Edgar Kaiser was building the Grand Coulee Dam in the state of Washington. This massive undertaking was financed out of public monies and employed large numbers of construction workers. Kaiser asked Garfield to create a program of health care for the workers and their families. This program was jointly paid for by employee and employer contributions, and it was considered a great success.

Kaiser Industries did not specialize only in dam construction. During World War II, it built cargo and troop carriers, popularly known as liberty ships. In 1942, this massive effort employed 90,000 workers in the San Francisco Bay area. Garfield was once again called upon to create a new program. After the war, the shipyards were closed and workers were dispersed. Garfield was left with a substantial group medical practice and a few thousand patients still employed by Kaiser Industries. Rather than reduce the size of the practice, he sought to keep it going by soliciting subscribers throughout the community, depending mainly on referrals (Cutting, 1971: 19). This recruitment drive was successful enough to keep the Kaiser Permanente program going. Still known by the name of the original employer (and the site of one of his cement factories), it had 970,000 members in several states in 1970. By 1998, according to its home page on the World Wide Web, it had programs in 19 states and the District of Columbia, serving 9.1 million people, and making Kaiser Permanente one of the largest HMOs in the country and, without doubt, the nation's largest nonprofit HMO.

A similar program, the Health Insurance Program or HIP, was created in New York City in the 1940s, primarily for municipal employees. Kaiser and HIP became the models for creating financial incentives for the health maintenance organizations found in federal legislation enacted in 1973. The formation of HMOs was supported through planning grants for medical groups and loans to cover losses during the early period when subscribers were being acquired. In addition, through this legislation companies with 25 or more employees are required to offer what is called "group-practice" services if they have group health insurance as a fully or partially paid fringe benefit, provided an approved HMO is available in the community where the corporation is located. This enabling legislation initially created legal problems, some having to do with the right of a union to bargain collectively over the fringe benefits available to members, and others having to do with the costs involved in meeting federal guidelines for planning grants and loans. Yet from these humble beginnings and with encouragement from government-employed health policy experts, the groundwork was established for the vast changes in health care delivery we are now experiencing.

MANAGED CARE EXPLAINED

Because it is based on rationing of services, managed care must get providers to agree to do only what is medically necessary. This restricts the autonomy of the professional, but it is supposed to be based on outcome studies that show the efficacy of interventions. Ideally, peer review determines what is permitted and what is not, and the decision to restrict access is not made by administrators who are untrained in medical matters. The creators of contemporary managed care plans sought to eliminate the anarchy of the medical workplace, with doctors evaluating, testing, and treating in many different ways. The goal of rationing is to eliminate ineffective procedures and unnecessary treatment, especially if it is very costly. According to the founders of managed care, this goal can be accomplished only through the participation of providers under the same management.

Providers are linked directly to the plans that agree to deliver all medical and health services to a subscriber. Uniformity of services is necessary in order to keep costs down and the plan, or health maintenance organization, can deliver the services at the rate they charge their customers or subscribers. Health plans hire actuaries to figure out what it will cost to deliver services to a given population, the sick as well as the healthy. Plans are capitalized to meet state insurance commission requirements so that rationing or the closing of the doors of the HMO does not occur because the plan simply miscalculated its expenditures in covering lives. While most of the original health maintenance organizations were nonprofit, this is no longer the case. Health plans are part of the commercial free enterprise system as well as run by organizations like Kaiser Permanente, Puget Sound, and Blue Cross/Blue Shield. The plan makes profits when the monetary value of the resources expended is less than the revenues taken in to cover the lives of subscribers and their dependents. In financial terms, what is expended on patient care is known as the medical-loss ratio. The value of the stock of a publicly offered HMO may plunge when the news gets out that a great many more patients were hospitalized during the last quarter of the year than was anticipated (Freudenheim, 1996). These losses reverberate in the financial markets because of the nature of financing health care in for-profit HMOs.

Whether profit making or nonprofit, the plan is paid upfront and it must live within the budget of what it takes in when it contracts to provide all medical and health services to a subscriber and dependents. Individuals who are covered by the plan pay a capitation fee, a fixed amount that provides medical services for a given period of time, regardless of the frequency of use, rather than paying fees for each service delivered. It is this capitation, or prepayment, that creates an incentive on the part of the providers to be cost conscious. A change in the composition of the patients recruited to the plan, known as the "case mix," can throw off the predicted service utilization.

Plans try to get as many healthy patients in their plans as they can so they can deliver services at the lowest cost possible. Patients are also recruited on the basis of a contract that stresses cost containment. Under capitation, they agree to use only the panel of doctors made available by the plan. In exchange for this agreement, they have no deductible payments before their insurance becomes activated. The co-payments they make when using the doctor are very modest—usually under $10 per visit.

Providers are paid on either a capitation basis if they are primary care providers, or, sometimes on a discounted fee-for-service basis. Under capitation, patients are encouraged to go as frequently as they want, while providers attempt to discourage unnecessary visits. Plans often feature many preventive services in order to avoid more expensive treatment. Providers who deliver primary care under capitation are encouraged to see the patients as infrequently as possible, to limit testing, and to make as few referrals to specialists as they can since they assume some financial risk. Providers who are paid on a fee-for-service basis are giving deep discounts to the plans they belong to and often have part of their fees withheld until an audit agrees that the actual visit rate and use of tests and other resources are within expected limits.

Sometimes the rules are suspended in recognition of unusual circumstances. If physicians have a disproportionately sick panel of patients, they may not be judged the same way as all other primary care providers; or some formula adjusted for adverse risk may be introduced to make comparisons possible with other doctors.

When hospitalization is needed, the patients must go to the hospitals that the plan approves of because it has contracts with these hospitals. The contract usually calls for the hospital to give a deep discount to the plan because it guarantees the hospital that a certain number of beds will be occupied. Discounting is also required of other suppliers such as pharmaceutical houses or surgical supply companies.

The new way of delivering care, through health maintenance organizations, has turned health care into a purchasable commodity. Moreover, it is produced in a more uniform and controlled work environment where there is little room for teaching and research—two of the missions of medicine, along with patient care. Each health maintenance organization is attempting to deliver a standardized product that would be recognizable by patients anywhere. In turn, the increasing emphasis on rationing makes it difficult for a patient to have any control in the marketplace. Since each plan is different, consumers cannot easily make careful comparisons. Moreover, consumers do not have the expertise that benefits officers in large corporations, through training and experience, have to make comparisons as to which is the better value.

HMOs operate according to standard business practices. As is the philosophy of American manufacturing, managers exhibit autocratic behavior in the workplace, and in turn, there is a kind of anarchy in the marketplace as the plans increasingly try to outdo each other in claiming they are the best. The advertisements for HMOs are starting to look like automobile ads, and this is not an accident since the marketing of these health plans has become similar to marketing any mass-produced product in the United States.

How did it come to be that managed care is now the *plat de jour* in American health care? The table has been set by the large multinational corporations that have become intolerant of the continued rise in the cost of health care in a system of third-party payment. There are now almost 60 million covered lives in HMOs and almost every group benefit package purchased by employers and paid for jointly by employees and employers has managed care features to reduce the use of health care services. For example, a benefits plan that allows the person covered to go directly to a specialist for a consultation will still require prior authorization if that specialist decides it is in the patient's best interest to remove a gall bladder. This particular kind of utilization review emanates from Medicare hospital regulations, which were enacted by Congress so it would be possible to identify providers who were hospitalizing patients unnecessarily. What all forms of utilization review do is to establish a prior constraint on providers, making it less likely they will perform an expensive procedure unnecessarily. MCO spokespeople regard these restraints on professionals as not only a form of cost containment but also a promotion of quality assurance since patients cannot benefit from an unnecessary procedure. In fact, many procedures, particularly surgery, involve risks to patients, sometimes resulting in injury or death. Other forms of quality assurance, such as encouraging immunization for children or Pap smears for women at appropriate intervals, are also promoted as the kind of preventions or early detections of disease that only MCOs are able to do well. This means that MCOs and their public relations units claim that they offer the best indemnity-based fee-for-service medicine in any comparison of performing preventive interventions.

With the exception of prior authorization to do an expensive procedure, the original form of financing health care in the United States, fee-for-service, still is reproduced in the encounter between a patient and a doctor outside of the HMO. Some existing plans, called preferred provider organizations (PPO), continue to use the fee-for-service system but limit the person covered to their list of providers. Patients can go to a specialist without seeing a generalist first and the providers on the list agree to give a deep discount to the plan. Furthermore, members pay a smaller co-payment when they use a physician who participates in the plan. At the end of 1995, the AAHP estimated that 91 million enrollees and dependents were in PPOs, an increase of 12 million from 1994.

Americans continue to be very price sensitive when it comes to health care. What managed care in its various forms has accomplished is the introduction of new reward systems for physicians and hospitals, and consumers as well, making it possible to deliver services at lower costs. These are significantly different ways of paying the doctor than are found in the American fee-for-service system. Each method of paying for medical services has incentives to providers and patients to do certain things and avoid other things. The fee-for-service system *without* third-party payment kept the charges down because physicians were afraid to scare away patients with high fees. Patients, in turn, were careful users of the system because their post-taxes' income went to pay for services. Besides, many of the encounters with physicians before the advent of antibiotics, such as penicillin, did not produce decisive interventions. The technology of medicine did not begin to get sophisticated until the 1950s. Consequently, most encounters with providers were not very expensive.

For those who could afford them as a regular source of care, before the widespread adoption of indemnity insurance in the 1960s, doctors were attentive, courteous, and warm. In an age where physicians depended on a limited market for their services, they had to demonstrate their devotion to the few patients they had. They wished to retain patients as much as possible and they wanted their patients to say good things about them in their neighborhoods, churches, and clubs. By keeping their fees low, doctors sought to cast as wide a net as possible to capture paying patients. In fact, general practitioners were reluctant to part with a patient through a referral to a specialist if they felt they could continue to help. Naturally, specialists knew this and expressed a great deal of gratitude for a referral because it was so hard won.

These arrangements worked to establish medicine as the major provider of health care services to the middle classes in the United States and to promote the development of the modern acute-care voluntary hospital as we know it today (Rosenberg, 1987). By the 1930s this system was threatened as the middle class's purchasing power declined. During the Great Depression patients could pay neither their hospital nor their doctor bills. First, in order to keep voluntary hospital beds filled and their doors open, group hospital insurance policies were underwritten and premiums collected from subscribers. Usually these policies were available to a work force that expected to be steadily employed, such as school teachers. Blue Cross hospital insurance was developed by the hospital industry itself as a way to keep generating income during those gloomy days. What worked in a mutually advantageous way for provider and consumer alike during hard times was even more popular during good times when more Americans wished to share in what became known in our popular culture as the "good life." However, first they were used as a way of keeping valued workers happy. Health insurance policies were offered as an across-the-board fringe benefit during World War II when wage and price freezes, compounded by a labor shortage, made it hard to retain employees without offering some reward. Then, during the postwar 1940s and 1950s, an era of substantial increases in real earnings and high progressive taxation, unionized workers sought to gain health benefits in collective bargaining agreements, sometimes in preference to increases in wages, because they were considered to be untaxed income.

The health insurance industry was off and running now and health care providers were beneficiaries; first, hospital bills were paid by insurance policies; and it was not too long before major medical care was also covered by indemnification policies. Benefits permitted potential patients and their providers to interact more; some of the real financial barriers to receiving medical care had been broken.

Insurance had major consequences in changing the behavior of patients and their doctors. Known as third-party payers, private insurance coverage made it possible for patients to seek doctors with great frequency, resulting in larger patient panels and more appointments per day. In fact, under these new financial conditions, which produced more patient volume, general practitioners were less reluctant to refer to specialists. The presence of coverage enhanced doctor-patient contact. For patients, insurance protected their assets since their medical bills were paid by third parties and they became less price sensitive. At the other end of the relationship, doctors found increased access generated more revenues; and since their operating costs were more or less fixed, it meant more income, both relatively and absolutely, as each additional patient seen during the day became an increasingly profitable consultation. Moreover, access to specialists was no longer restricted by economic considerations. Each referral was less essential to their practices, but as with general practitioners, it was also more economically valuable than in the past. The advent of Medicare and Medicaid merely accelerated processes of growth in the industry rather than initiating them.

The explosion in health care inflation was exacerbated by the growth of technology, generated by new markets for its use. Third-party payment made consumers less price conscious in the health care marketplace. The development of new technology means greater profits for the manufacturers so long as their products are accepted as a standard tool in the doctor's arsenal. It is precisely because physicians in fee-for-service medicine became partners in owning this technology that health policy analysts and benefits officers became unwilling to underwrite the seemingly unlimited inflation in health care services.

The plan is fairly simple: Manufacturers of diagnostic equipment, monitoring devices, and pharmaceuticals all need to get the *real* consumer, i.e., the physician, to use their products. Getting these products accepted involves efforts of persuasion comparable to the selling to any target audience of consumers. The manufacturers do have a built-in advantage, given the nature of fee-for-service medical practice in the United States. Physicians are more highly rewarded, both materially and professionally, by performing procedures rather than engaging in educational efforts with patients. Third-party payers regard these procedures as more complex than patient education and reimburse claims more handsomely when technology is used. In addition, the more procedures performed with *physician-owned* diagnostic equipment, the more financially rewarding these procedures are. Recent studies point to the differences in the use of diagnostic equipment according to ownership by the examining physician. Moreover, the task can usually be delegated to a technician who can gain increasing proficiency at doing these tasks unsupervised while the physician can be doing other things. Reporting in 1991, the Florida Health Care Cost Containment Board, a state agency, found that when doctors owned their own laboratories, almost twice as many tests were performed for each patient as at other laboratories. Similar results were found in this comprehensive Florida study of frequency of scheduled visits to physical therapy centers that were owned in joint ventures by doctors (*New York Times*, August 11, 1991: E9). According to the report, 45 percent of the state's doctors were involved in such arrangements. Over 90 percent of the diagnostic imaging centers in Florida were wholly or partly owned by doctors.

The Florida report also concluded that the poor and rural residents did not have improved access to these diagnostic and clinical services despite their proliferation around the state. This kind of finding is not limited to areas where senior citizens abound. Around the same time, a more systematic statewide study of almost 38,000 patients at 100 hospitals, reported in the *Journal of the American Medical Association*, found that patients with the same symptoms receive more diagnostic testing when they are covered by insurance than when they are not (Wenneker, 1990). Massachusetts patients with chest pains or circulatory problems who were insured were more likely to be diagnosed or treated for heart disease than those patients without insurance or those who were covered by Medicaid. Equipment and staff time is sometimes used selectively so that the procedures ordered up will yield greater revenues. Similarly, patients who are Medicaid eligible yield lower returns for the same diagnostic procedures as those who are insured or covered by the Medicare program and, consequently, receive less testing.

Paralleling the extension of technology as part of the relationship with patients was the development of life-extending technology for those near death. Respirators were originally designed for and used with patients who had lung surgery, allowing these organs to recover slowly. Additional uses were found in intensive care units for this equipment as patients who were in critical condition, with multiple organ failures, were placed on respirators.

Following the scholarly exposé in a major medical journal on involuntary clinical experimentation initiated by Beecher (1966), in which he cited numerous studies where patients never gave informed consent to participate in dangerous experiments, federal legislators and patient rights advocates questioned how much choice patients had in undergoing clinical procedures or treatment regimens that might be futile or invasive, or have adverse side effects. The ensuing development of informed consent for standard clinical care followed on the heels of similar protocols to protect the rights of subjects in experiments. It is not surprising that consumers began to wonder whether they were being told everything or whether doctors knew how to communicate with patients. However, it was undoubtedly the crisis of rising costs of health care that spurred medical ethicists to begin to see that patients had little choice to refuse these invasive procedures with questionable efficacy.

Now device manufacturers face harder times, as the HMOs take a close look at how much they need in the way of expensive technology. Where once technology was moved quickly into office- and hospital-based practice, today, providers and payers want to know what is necessary and what works (Borzo, 1996: 4). The reduction in fee-for-service medicine, combined with third-party payment, is finally reducing the demand for new technology.

When third-party payment augments but does not replace the classic fee-for-service relationship between doctors and patients, it still means some out-of-pocket costs for routine office visits. The concept of insurance was a way to protect against major economic catastrophes that could befall a family, such as those resulting from the death of the major wage earner, the loss of a home, or the loss of a business. Some consumers and a few providers became concerned about the high cost of services rendered. Models for how to rein in out-of-pocket expenditures did exist, although the American Medical Association severely disapproved of doctors who worked for a salary—the keystone of the first-generation HMOs that provided comprehensive care for a single fee paid up front. Kaiser and other early health maintenance organizations delivered good services at a moderate cost to the membership. In so doing, consumers "locked in" their health care costs for an entire year through this prepayment arrangement with specific providers. Not only were doctors' services available under these plans, but hospital care was also provided for a single fee, with the provider assuming the financial risk if there was an unexpected utilization.

Ever since the 1960s employers have been concerned about controlling their expenditures for health care and have looked for ways of avoiding increases in the costs of services. In addition, consumers have tried to lock in their annual costs for health care. Today, in HMO programs, a group of doctors, including specialists, provide all the medical specialties and services by contract to a number of patients who will be cared for, no matter how frequently or infrequently they use the services. Additionally, hospital-based services are part of the contracted benefits and are pre-arranged by contracts between HMOs and hospitals or by outright purchase or building of hospitals exclusively dedicated to care for subscribers.

Skills learned in business schools and cost-based planning drive HMOs today. Contemporary HMOs are less likely to be staffed by salaried physicians who work in HMO-owned offices and hospitals and are more likely to be part of a network of providers. The over-capacity of the hospital system has made it possible for HMOs to drive hard bargains with community hospitals and academic medical centers to admit their patients, when appropriate, at well below the rate charged the indemnity insurance companies.

Cost-consciousness is raised to a high art in managed care organizations. Managed care will pay for low-cost preventive medicine, early detection and treatment of disease, and health promotion activities such as smoking-cessation programs. Marketing is directed toward those who are healthy, focusing on health promotion activities such as discounted memberships in fitness centers, rather than showing how well they care for stroke victims. It limits benefits in instances where decision makers regard the care as pure comfort and not always medically necessary, as in the case of hospital stays for psychiatric care and unlimited psychotherapy. Care coordination for complex cases may also be part of an HMO's way of making sure that physicians do not order unnecessary care. Service substitution also takes place, as when nurse practitioners and physician associates provide primary care under the supervision of a physician, or when outpatient care is given instead of hospitalizing the patient.

In sum, managed care means that the providers are watched carefully to make sure that they do not provide unnecessary care. Medical care is also rationed through prior authorization mechanisms, a form of micromanagement that professionals thoroughly resent. Even before a sick person gets to the point of needing some expensive specialty-based procedure, the primary care provider is performing gatekeeping functions in the HMO, making sure that when a specialist is seen it is truly for something that the primary care provider cannot do.

By stressing prevention and early intervention, HMOs are able to deliver comprehensive services at reasonable costs. Certainly HMOs have an admirable record with regard to childhood immunizations. Yet there is another side to medical practice and that involves care when you are seriously ill. Critics of HMOs suggest that seeing fewer specialists is not necessarily a good thing, especially if you suffer from a serious chronic condition or disability. Moreover, in many HMOs, specialty services may be available at "centers of excellence" but they are not accessible because they are not near where subscribers live. Plan financial agents may develop contracts with facilities that provide deep discounts, but because they deal with rare diseases they may be far from a given patient's home community and therefore cannot always accommodate routine family needs, including being able to hold on to one's job. One North Carolina family underwent total disruption when a child required bone marrow transplants, only available under the plan in Baltimore, Maryland (Weston and Lauria, 1996). As Harry and Louise might have said in their famous 1993 commercial for the status quo during the health insurance industry's clever battle against health care reform, "There's got to be a better way."

SAVINGS, SAVINGS, SAVINGS

The success of managed care in convincing employers that they will cut their costs for fringe benefits has meant that there are few straight indemnity plans left in the group insurance market. By 1997, employer-sponsored conventional insurance without precertification requirements for expensive procedures, the most elementary form of utilization review, comprised no more than 2 percent of the private insurance market. Conventional plans with precertification amounted to only 16 percent of the employer-sponsored market (KPMG, 1998).

Savings are derived in managed care from providing fewer services and getting them at lower prices. This usually is interpreted by advocates for managed care as meaning that inappropriate and unnecessary services are eliminated when utilization review and active case management takes place. Incentive to do this kind of care to generate revenue, as was the case in a fee-for-service system, does not exist in managed care. Moreover, the purchasing power of HMOs means that they can get deep discounts from providers and let contracts that have providers assuming much or all of the financial risk for enrollees. Only those providers who are less costly and hopefully more efficient are selected to participate in an MCO.

There are also indirect savings generated when managed care penetrates a regional market. To compete, sellers of other forms of insurance will lower their prices to keep or gain market share. Comparisons of the costs of care delivery performed by health economists, in reviewed articles in journals and in publications of the Congressional Budget Office, show substantial savings in MCOs. Moreover, there is also a consensus among these researchers that there is a "spillover effect" in a regional market that impacts on traditional indemnity insurance costs (Health Economics Practice, 1998).

HEALTH CARE REFORM AND MANAGED CARE

Are we better off today, with managed care sweeping away indemnity coverage? Are vulnerable populations, particularly those with serious chronic illnesses and disabilities, well served by this transition in the way we pay for and organize health care services?

The market road to cutting costs in health care has done little to make the American citizen feel more secure, knowing that unregulated competition is in the driver's seat. Since 1992, with this enormous growth in HMO membership and the addition of managed care features to indemnity insurance policies, the public has not regarded these changes as beneficial. A public opinion poll conducted by the *New York Times* in June 1996—three and a half years into the Clinton administration and two years after the failure of health care reform legislation—nearly one-third of the 1,121 people surveyed (32 percent) said that health care had gotten worse since Mr. Clinton became president. Only 12 percent said it had gotten better (Wines and Pear, 1996: B8). The blame for decline in quality was laid at the doors of the big insurance companies and the big HMOs and not the president. The public got it right in saying that the failure to enact universal health insurance was due to the stonewalling of health care legislation by the Republicans in 1993 and 1994, as well as by the Republican Congress elected in 1994. The small business lobby was overjoyed that they did not get an employer mandate to provide insurance and the big corporations were happy to see their costs hold steady, if not decline. The result was that employees had fewer plans to choose from. The possible loss of choice of trusted providers, paradoxically, was the key fear among the public's refusal to buy into the Clintons' Health Security Act.

REFERENCES

American Association of Health Plans. 1996. *1995–1996 AAHP HMO and PPO Trends Report.* http://www.aahp.org/LI/RESEARCH

American Medical News. 1991. "HMOs successful in big cities, old markets." *American Medical News* (February 18): 33.

Beecher, H. K. 1966. "Consent in clinical experimentation: Myth and reality." *Journal of the American Medical Association* 195 (January 3): 34–35.

Borzo, G. 1996. "Managed care and technology assessment: Who should pay?" *Technology News* (March): 3–4.

Cutting, C. 1971. "Historical development and operating concepts." In Anne R. Somers, editor, *The Kaiser Permanente Medical Care Program.* New York: Commonwealth Fund.

Freeborn, D. K., and Pope, C. R. 1994. *Promise and Performance in Managed Care: The Prepaid Group Practice Model.* Baltimore: Johns Hopkins University Press.

Freudenheim, M. 1996. "Market place: HMOs are having trouble maintaining financial health." *New York Times* (June 19th): D12.

Health Economics Practice. 1998. "Impacts of four legislative provisions on managed care consumers: 1999–2003." Prepared for the American Association of Health Plans. Barents Group, Washington, DC.

Hoffman, C., Rice, D., and Sung, H. Y. 1996. "Persons with chronic conditions: Their prevalence and costs." *Journal of the American Medical Association* 276: 1473–1479.

Keene, C. 1971. "Kaiser Industries and Kaiser Permanente health care partnership." In Anne R. Somers, editor, *The Kaiser Permanente Medical Care Program*. New York: Commonwealth Fund.

KPMG. 1998. *Surveys of employer-sponsored health benefits*. New York: KPMG.

New York Times. 1991. "When doctors own their own labs." *New York Times* (August 11th): E9.

Rosenberg, C. 1987. *The Care of Strangers: The Rise of America's Hospital System*. New York: Basic Books.

Schlesinger, M., and Mechanic, D. 1993. "Challenges for managed competition from chronic illness." *Health Affairs* 12 (Supplement): 123–137.

U.S. Office of Technology Assessment. 1986. *Nurse Practitioners, Physician Assistants and Certified Nurse-Midwives: A Policy Analysis*. Technology Case Study 37. Washington, DC: Government Printing Office.

Wenneker, M. B. 1990. "The association of payer with utilization of cardiac procedures in Massachusetts." *Journal of the American Medical Association* 264 (10) (September 12th): 1255–1260.

Weston, B., and Lauria, M. 1996. "Patient advocacy in the 1990s." *New England Journal of Medicine* (February 22nd): 334–335.

Wines, M., and Pear, R. 1996. "President finds benefits in defeat on health care." *New York Times* (July 30th): A1, B8.

4

A Cost-Driven Delivery System
and People with Disabilities

Ever since the middle of the 1980s, there has been a persistent concern among health care policy experts that the often lifelong medical needs of people with disabilities generate serious financial problems for themselves and their families (Anderson, 1985). This concern was spurred on by the practice of insurance underwriters of using experience rating rather than community rating as a way of determining the premium for a group or individual health insurance policy. In other words, insurers avoided risk by not covering people with pre-existing conditions or not covering expenses related to care for those conditions. What went on was a practice known as "cherry picking" or "cream skimming." The healthy were insurable because the costs to indemnify their care were predicted to be far less than those of people with serious chronic illnesses or disabilities. A moderate number of articulate people came forth to tell their stories of exclusion from private insurance coverage, either for themselves or their children.

At the same time, national probability studies of utilization of services showed serious underuse for individuals without insurance coverage. Individuals without health plan benefits had limited access to care. Often families had incomes that made them ineligible for means-tested benefits programs such as Medicaid but could not afford private insurance. The results of such situations were highly predictable: Individuals with the same conditions or limitations without insurance made fewer physician visits than those with insurance. Moreover, with or without insurance, out-of-pocket expenses for those considered in poor health were 2.5 times greater than for those in good health (National Center for Health Statistics, 1987). These tales of financial anxiety, compounding concerns about access to care, later helped to promote the brief but failed campaign for health care reform initiated by the Clintons in 1993.

The transition to managed care, largely a result of business decisions in the corporate world, produced a new issue. Policy makers continued their concern about access, but they worried more about stinting on services in managed care than the impact on people with disabilities of not having health insurance or having heavy out-of-pocket expenditures. The growth of managed care captured the attention of every commentator on health care in the nation, including advocates for the disabled.

The shift of concern began in the 1990s. The year 1993 marked the first time that the *majority* of employees and their families with health plan coverage were in managed care plans (Iglehart, 1994: 1167). By 1995, five states had implemented the Federal Health Care Financing Administration's Section 1115 waivers—allowing states to move from legally guaranteed benefits to Medicaid beneficiaries. The state waivers are attempts to contain expenditures through conversion of Medicaid coverage and service delivery to managed care. In the same year, three more states were approved but had not yet implemented the waivers of the Federal Health Care Financing Administration (Holahan et al., 1995). The disruptive effects of these changes in Medicaid were noted in early observations regarding the quality of care. Buchanan et al. (1992) reported that special needs populations sometimes found it difficult to identify Medicaid managed care plans that had experience dealing with the special health conditions of their clients.

Who are the winners and who are the losers, following this conversion in financing and organization of the health care delivery system? In anticipation of some of the major financially driven components of managed care, Andrew Batavia, former executive director of the Federal National Council on Disability, concluded that "cost containment provisions that focus on the provider, such as global budgeting and managed competition, will adversely affect disabled people if providers do not have adequate incentives to meet these people's needs" (1993: 41).

The issue of stinting was framed by contemporary students of HMOs. Freund and Lewit (1993) note that there are particular concerns about the negative effects of managed care for vulnerable populations:

plans with strong incentives to reduce utilization might limit services needed by children . . . whose medical care might be difficult or costly to deliver. Special concern is raised because primary care physicians who are at risk financially may face disincentives to refer their chronically ill patients to specialists, to rehabilitation, or to extended psychiatric care or the like. (100)

FUNCTION DRIVES STRUCTURE

In a system designed to contain costs, the big losers are the big users, whether the focus is on providers or patients. It has become common knowledge among students of health care systems that roughly 80 percent of the expenditures go to 20 percent or fewer of those covered, whether financing occurred through Medicare, Medicaid, or private insurance. Managed care continues the tradition of avoiding financial risks started in the 1980s with indemnity insurers. HMOs love healthy patients and like to keep them healthy. They even go out of their way to recruit among the healthy, offering discounts at fitness centers to attract those without limitations in function and without disabilities or secondary conditions that need attention. This is clearly a form of risk avoidance through marketing since they do not recruit with equal passion on the pages of periodicals that reach large numbers of people with disabilities, for example, the American Association of Retired Persons' stately *Modern Maturity* or the wickedly funny *Disability Rag*.

I have no doubt that more integrated services, built around care coordination, would be of great benefit to people with disabilities. However, there are several structured outcomes in the way services are planned that create risks for people with disabilities in managed care settings. Some of these concerns would also apply to indemnity health coverage. However, as pure indemnity insurance seems to be a thing of the past, the advocates in the disability community have focused their anger at both the changes wrought by managed care and the ongoing lack of accommodation to people with disabilities. There is even a current effort by the Consortium on Disability and Health to show through litigation that HMOs are in violation of the Americans with Disabilities Act because of their failure to accommodate people with disabilities.

There may even be no conscious intent of excluding the disabled from health care according to policy. However, the MCO way of organizing services leaves people with disabilities at a structured disadvantage. The playing field, in other words, remains metaphorically an uphill one for the disabled. First, there is the reliance on the principle of service substitution and restriction, which may be worthwhile in general but may be risky for people with disabilities. Moreover, since the consumer advisory boards of HMOs and other types of plans do not consist of consumers but often benefits officers from local employers, it is not easy to communicate the special needs of people with disabilities. It would be a valuable way to enhance consumer satisfaction if HMOs went out of their way to recruit advisory board members who had serious chronic illnesses and disabilities. Their points of view could lead to policy accommodations within what is often a rigid structure of service delivery.

HMOs traditionally undertake efforts to build health care services around the primary care provider, creating less reliance on specialists. From a cost containment perspective, this may be a good idea. Reducing unnecessary visits to specialists, and consequently unnecessary diagnostic testing, saves money because it is proven that specialists do more testing than primary care providers. Sometimes MCOs go further and substitute nurse practitioners and physician assistants for the usual primary care providers—internal medicine generalists, family physicians, and pediatricians—since these new middle-level practitioners can do excellent work in prevention and early detection of disease; and, of course, they are less expensive to employ because they can be compensated at a lower rate than physicians. Other forms of substitution involve using adult specialists, for example, a neurologist to provide health care for children who might benefit from seeing a pediatric subspecialist, such as a developmental pediatrician.

There is no doubt that health plans are arranged to discourage the use of specialty care. In a systematic review of recent studies related to the influence of MCOs on physician referral, Grembowski, Cook, Patrick, and Roussel (1998) found that patients in plans that only pay for network specialists or where the network contains a smaller percentage of specialists have a lower probability of referral. Utilization management policy often requires prior authorization for referrals or approval for only one visit rather than multiple visits. Sometimes approval for referral must come from the group practice's medical director rather than the primary care provider (PCP). Close review of referral practices discourages PCPs from making referrals as well as putting forth financial disincentives. Patients who have to pay large out-of-pocket costs, such as for mental health services, are also less likely to use those providers.

Second, there is a practice in most MCOs of limiting access to ongoing ancillary services, such as speech, physical, and occupational therapies. These therapies will not make most people with disabilities better but they are needed to maintain current functioning. Health insurance companies and MCOs have developed definitions of medical necessity that work against people with disabilities because they use "cure" as the justification for treatment. While improvement may be slight from a cure perspective, there may be a reduction in limitations so that a person with a disability can have a better quality of life, including being more productive. Sometimes the therapies are approved, but there are upper limits on how many visits will be paid for by the plan.

Third, there is also a related issue with regard to medical necessity. People with disabilities, especially children, may have conditions for which there are no official designations found in such guidebooks as the *Ninth International Classification of Disease* (ICD-9). Limits on an individual's functioning exist even when providers cannot make a clear identification of etiology or even a designation of the exact condition. Payment for care is often tied to an ICD-9 code and failure on the part of a provider to use a code does not mean that there is no need for intervention, only confusion as to what to call it.

Fourth, there is a similar constraint exercised when durable medical equipment (DME) is not covered by an MCO or is covered basically to make it possible to acquire a prosthetic or other form of assistance that only makes for limited improvement in mobility, and consequently, minor gain in the quality of life. It should be noted that traditional indemnity insurance was no more generous than MCOs when it came to paying for DME. However, the disability community has used this issue to point out how unfair both financing systems are and to get better benefits when it came to coverage for DME.

Criticism of the entire American health care delivery system from a disability perspective has been building with the multinational participation in the ongoing revisions of the 1980 *International Classification of Impairments, Disabilities, and Handicaps* (ICIDH-2). The new attempt to create a common language for functioning and disablement has morphed into *The International Classification of Impairments, Activities and Participation*, but it is still known as ICIDH-2. Produced by the World Health Organization and scheduled for completion in 2000, the objective of this effort is to better define: (1) the need for health care and related services; and (2) health outcomes in terms of body, person, and social functioning. In so doing, the planners of this ambitious effort seek a common framework for research, clinical work, and social policy as well as ensuring the cost-effective provision and management of health care and related services.

Briefly, to improve the lives and functioning of people with disabilities, the ICIDH-2 managers argue, we need to get away from the medical classification of diagnoses since they alone do not predict what kinds of interventions are needed. The biopsychosocial model advocated as appropriate for dealing with disability has three parts. First, there are impairment interventions—medical actions to deal with the impairment and preventive interventions to avoid activity limitations. Second, activity limitation interventions are rehabilitative, including the provision of assistive technology and personal assistance to mitigate activity limitation. Third, participation restriction interventions seek through public education, legal protections, and architechtural design to accomodate activity limitations.

According to this model, the ICIDH-2 (World Health Organization, 1998) creates three parallel classifications related to level of functioning: impairment, activities, and participation.

- *Impairment* is a loss or abnormality of body structure or a physiological or psychological function (e.g., hearing loss, loss of limb).

- An *activity* is the nature and extent of functioning at the level of the person. Activities may be limited in nature, duration, and quality (e.g., taking care of oneself, performing the activities required of a job).

- *Participation* is the nature and extent of a person's involvement in life situations in relation to Impairment, Activities, Health Conditions, and Contextual Factors. Participation may be restricted in nature, duration, and quality (e.g., being employed, participating in community activities).

In sum, this classification system calls attention to services that would permit individuals to personally engage in instrumental and self-care activities of daily living and participate in conventional settings.

There are many steps that need to be mastered to gain the desired outcomes of self-care and the performance of the tasks associated with employment. Intermediate objectives for the rehabilitation of a stroke victim, for example, regaining intelligible speech or walking, need to be carefully established as a milestone on the way to greater independence and productivity. It also should be noted that results on this level may not come about in every case without expending substantial resources or allowing for extra time.

Medical rehabilitation experts have sought to advance outcomes research in the field of disability (Fuhrer, 1997). The National Center for Medical Rehabilitation Research has begun to focus on the problem of how to convince payers that what is done to assist people with disabilities does make a difference. Many of the highly individualized therapies and treatment plans undertaken to improve, restore, or retain independence are vulnerable to cost cutters working for managed care organizations. Because of the small number of subjects available for controlled research trials, there are methodologic difficulties in designing randomized controlled studies. Fuhrer and his colleagues presented papers at a 1994 conference that featured rehabilitation practices that could be justified because they produced measurable results. When funders became the controlling interest, whether private or public, they initiated a race among rehabilitation providers to show that what they did was not only worthwhile but could be quantified.

Fifth, the financing of access to enabling services has been particularly weak in MCOs. In some ways the disability community is using the transition to managed care to call attention to the costly services that they must have in order to get to the doctor and/or simply get around in the home. Transportation is a major out-of-pocket expense for individuals with disabilities, including visits to doctors or therapists. Ambulette services are expensive, and people with disabilities are also frequent users of health services, a factor that can make for multiple usage during the year. For those with more severe limitations in ADL, there is also a need for personal assistance, a service that is not covered very well by the private insurance system. In addition, financing of translators for the deaf or those with major hearing impairments can be expensive, and the MCO is not likely to pay for them.

Finally, some of these changes are criticized because the new system does not guarantee access to the same providers who the person with a disability saw in the past. When picking a primary care provider, it may not be possible to select someone with experience in working with people with disabilities or the particular disability of concern. Moreover, even when a person with a disability seems to be willing to try a new provider, there is still no guarantee of finding someone with experience. Primary care providers are not always trained in giving care to the disabled portion of the population.

Little training and few patients with disabilities may be a way of asking for trouble. Pushing generalists beyond their competencies goes against ingrained professionalism, that is, physicians know the limits of their knowledge and skills. Providers with little experience may overlook something of great importance that needs an intervention. Some advocates have argued that *all* primary care providers need intensive as well as extensive training in caring for people with disabilities. In that way the goal of inclusion can be obtained when getting excellent medical care. However, if people with disabilities were randomly disbursed among all the primary care providers (PCP) in all the managed care plans, each PCP would care for very few with the same chronic condition. Few of the benefits of repetition would be available in those medical encounters.

There is no consensus in the disability community about whether it is better for all primary care providers to have a modicum of training in caring for the disabled or if a few should become exceptionally knowledgeable so they can be the physicians to whom a person with a disability is routed. This lack of information calls out for a controlled experiment with random assignment to experimental and control groups.

The civil rights goals of inclusion and integration march right up to the threshold of the doctor's examining room. Advocates expect equal treatment even when it may be unrealistic to suggest that all primary care providers will be, or should be, equally well trained in how to provide medical care for people with disabilities.

My own opinion is that having experience with people with disabilities is a distinct advantage in giving good care. Without that experience, even the best intentioned provider might overlook something of importance. It has been shown that cardiac artery bypass grafting (CABG) achieves better outcomes (i.e., lower mortality rates) with the more procedures the surgical unit does. This same logic should be applied to most medical encounters where the patient has some complex condition to which attention must be paid. Even something relatively simple, such as repair of a hernia, is performed more effectively and efficiently by a surgeon who exclusively does these operations, as at the Shouldice Hospital of Toronto (Gawande, 1998).

In an evolving managed care system, the training of physicians in practice to deal with disability has not been clearly defined. There are two possible approaches to rectify the problem of providers lacking the clinical skills, knowledge, and communications skills to appropriately manage the care of individuals with disabilities and help their families or care givers.

The first is to introduce the issues to physicians-in-training, beginning when they are medical students and continuing through their residency training, so that they have a significant exposure to the diagnosis and treatment of children and adults with disabilities. Thus far, only board certification requirements in pediatrics demand at least a one-month training experience in developmental and behavioral pediatrics. The second approach is through continuing education of physicians currently enrolled in provider organizations, along with nurse practitioners and others serving HMOs as primary care providers. This would require reaching out by academic medical centers to assure the availability of satisfactory continuing education experiences.

Briefly, this training should deal with how to identify disabilities early, and when and how to make appropriate referrals for interdisciplinary diagnosis and treatment. It should enhance knowledge of the importance of inclusion of the available community resources (and just what these services are) and should provide reliable information about the prognosis and the anticipated life cycle of individuals with different types and degrees of disability, as well as impart a clear understanding of families' needs, largely through consumer input.

A managed care pediatric practice in Arizona provides some reassuring evidence about the way primary care providers can deal effectively with children with disabilities. Phoenix Pediatrics has been serving children with special health care needs on a capitated basis for 12 years. Of the 30,000 children in the practice, 2,000 have substantial special health care needs, including children with developmental disabilities, attention deficit disorder, cerebral palsy, and epilepsy, as well as children who require gastrostomy tube feedings or who are tracheostomy- or home ventilator- dependent (Brooks, 1997: 362).

Through experience with this special needs population, physicians have learned to train parents to do many procedures at home, thus reducing hospitalization and office visits. Sophisticated discharge planning along with intensive case management has also made a difference in resource utilization. Physicians have learned these case management skills on-the-job. They have also come to rely on medical management via telephone calls.

The physicians have to devise their own data collection schemes since there are no established measures of quality ambulatory care for special needs children. Using this information, and depending on the number of disabilities that a child has, they negotiate better than standard rates with the MCOs in the Phoenix area.

STANDARDIZATION

Designers of managed care organizations believe that medical utilization can be shifted to less costly yet more effective care and that medical outcomes can be significantly improved in the process. Fewer unnecessary procedures may result in less death and injury to patients. Less time in the hospital may mean less exposure to infections that travel from patient to care giver to yet another patient. Less may be more in the medical arena. Not every old practice is worthwhile and not every new practice has a payoff.

The development of clinical practice guidelines can get all doctors on the same page, so to speak, encouraging them to manage the care of their patients in similar ways. These guidelines are developed through consensus among clinicians with a great deal of experience caring for individuals with particular chronic diseases. Guidelines are created first for conditions that have high prevalence rates and involve costly interventions. While driven by cost containment, there are also positive patient care outcomes to consider.

Disease management programs aim to use information collected from patients to get them to adhere to drug and dietary regimens. In addition, clinical and laboratory reports also may be used to find out whether patient adherence has produced better utilization and clinical outcomes. Monitoring patients can have impressive payoffs for all concerned. When patients with heart failure were recently tracked at the Kaiser Permanent Medical Care Program of Northern California, the results showed fewer medical visits, emergency department visits, and hospital admissions. More important, symptoms declined in severity, including reductions in reported fatigue, shortness of breath, or discomfort in breathing while lying flat (West et al., 1997).

Similar kinds of disease management programs need to be developed to provide medical care for people with cerebral palsy, brain injury, and other disabilities. There is a dearth of practice guidelines in the field of disability as well as specific management programs with defined outcomes.

The process of delivering services to people with disabilities may be improved with standardization but accommodation is also needed. Two Chicago physicians, David Ebert and Paul Heckerling (1998), followed over 600 patients admitted to a general medical service at a university hospital. They wanted to find out what kinds of communication disabilities existed in this cohort and to determine whether special accommodations were necessary.

Simple functional assessments were made through consensus by the medical team. For example, patients were

> judged to have a serious communication disability if their vision was so poor that they were unable to read hospital consent forms or typical patient-education materials, even with their corrective lenses; if they could not understand shouted speech, even with their hearing aids; if they could not produce speech understandable to the medical team; or if they had altered mental states. (272–273)

Not surprising, given the epidemiology of disability presented in chapter 1, the authors found that almost 16 percent of their patients had severe disabilities affecting communication. Nine percent had altered mental states, 4.7 percent vision impairments, 2.8 percent speech impairments, and 0.5 percent hearing impairments. Affected patients were most likely to be older males. Communication disabilities were associated with such conditions as diabetic retinopathy, glaucoma, cataracts, strokes or other neuro-logic disorders, and head and neck cancers. Services to improve communi-cation are not often provided in health care settings. Increasingly, health care providers working with high patient loads may overlook important symptoms when dealing with patients with communication disabilities.

The growth of services for people with disabilities, especially in the field of developmental disabilities (with their early onset), has not been guided by any need to measure outcomes in terms of improvements in productivity or independence. Service providers, ever since efforts began in the 1970s to close the large and isolated institutions, have been guided by legally pro-tected principles of self-determination for consumers. This is particularly evident in the protections available for consumers to ensure that they es-tablish what it is they want in the way of individualized services. Providers' accepted practices may prove to be recondite in the face of changes im-posed by managed care organizations.

Standardization of health care for people with disabilities may be diffi-cult because of the idiosyncratic nature of these conditions. The methodol-ogy for the development of treatment plans—generated by clinical practice guidelines and medical outcomes research that deals with acute conditions or even chronic illness, such as heart failure—may not be ap-propriate for individuals with multiple diagnoses. This may be particularly evident for individuals with behavioral and intellectual deficits or some combination of the two.

Despite the extreme differences that can exist among individuals with the same disabilities, as well as conditions that baffle medical providers and limit the application of standardized practices through guidelines, there have been some substantial reports on the experiences of people with dis-abilities with HMOs.

Although only a small part of the population with disabilities qualifies for Medicare through participation in the Social Security Disability Insur-ance (SSDI) program or the Railroad Retirement program, the experiences of this population shed light on the advantages and disadvantages of HMO enrollment. First, SSDI and Railroad Retirement enrollees can be com-pared with elderly Medicare HMO members with regard to their satisfac-tions with services and problems in gaining access to services. Second, the SSDI and Railroad Retirement enrollees can be compared with those with similar entitlement status who do not join HMOs and get their medical care from Medicare providers in the fee-for-service system.

Whether functional limitations have an early onset or are derived later in life, they can, following medical examinations, create an official certifi-cation for individuals in contemporary American society, producing entitlements for those who are defined as disabled. Following a definition of disability that requires that there be found an inability to engage in substantial, gainful activity by reason of mental or physical impairment, nonelderly individuals cannot only receive monthly stipends for income support but can also become Medicare beneficiaries.

Predictably, an income maintenance program such as SSDI may be very important to disabled people who cannot work. Recent Harris Poll data indicate that "only 29 percent of disabled people of working age (18–64) work full or part-time, compared to 79 percent of the population in general" (Disability News Service, 1998: 3). This sample had annual incomes far below the elderly in the survey who had multiple sources of income beyond social security old age pensions. Pension eligibility is not likely to occur for the SSDI population, many of whom only have sporadic work experiences.

The members of the sample in the survey were varied as to the nature of their conditions, with many reporting more than one disorder, as can be seen in the following listing:

> Just under a third (31 percent) of those surveyed by the MCBS reported mental or psychiatric disorders, about half of whom (15 percent) said that this was their reason for becoming eligible. Among disabled Medicare beneficiaries, 38 percent reported hypertension, 35 percent arthritis, 23 percent health conditions other than angina pectoris or chronic heart disease (which accounted for another 13 percent), 21 percent partial paralysis, 19 percent mental retardation, and 18 percent emphysema and various other pulmonary diseases. (Gold et al., 1997: 152)

Like all individuals eligible for Medicare, the SSDI population can choose fee-for-service providers or an HMO for medical care. An analysis undertaken by staff at Mathematica Policy Research for the 1996 national Medicare Current Beneficiary Survey (MCBS) of 3,080 beneficiaries found that most of the disabled people enrolled in Medicare HMOs did not experience access problems. However, when compared to elderly Medicare HMO users, they did experience more problems getting care (Gold et al., 1997). (It is possible that HMOs are not as experienced in caring for this population as they are for the elderly; or, alternatively, since they became Medicare eligible at a relatively young age, they have more severe medical problems than the elderly.) The general level of satisfaction was high enough for 89 percent of the SSDI Medicare respondents in the survey to say that they would recommend their plan to a family member or friend.

We should recognize that people with disabilities, like everyone else, are concerned about the way out-of-pocket expenses have increased over the last two decades. Visiting the HMO primary care provider may not be as pleasant as seeing a doctor in fee-for-service medicine, but it does eliminate deductibles and downsizes co-payments to modest amounts, usually $10 or less. Moreover, a prescription plan for a patient taking expensive or multiple drug products can be a major money saver. Since the annual incomes of people with disabilities are significantly less than the incomes of the rest of population, the savings produced by HMO membership may be impressive for the consumer.

HMOs have been a form of affordable health care for those people with disabilities under age 65 who have Medicare coverage. They have joined in many areas where senior citizens were signed up for these managed care plans. However, in the last few years, HMOs have found that they can no longer make money by providing health care for the Medicare population. Changes in the rate structure found in the Balanced Budget Act of 1997 have led to the dumping of Medicare-eligible individuals back to fee-for-service care. Since Medicare does not cover many out-of-hospital services including prescriptions, the insurance industry, under congressional guidance, has developed a limited number of products to underwrite Medicare gap coverage, or "Medigap," as it is known.

At last look, insurance industry officials were afraid that people with disabilities would seek these policies once they were dropped from Medicare HMOs. The Medigap policies are sold at rates that are not based on actuarial calculations that include people with disabilities. Spokespeople for the Health Insurance Association of America have claimed that the disabled were "carved out" of Medigap coverage when Congress did not specifically include them. Initially, Clinton administration officials at the Health Care Financing Administration (HCFA) interpreted the rules about who can buy Medigap insurance differently than the industry, and a battle appeared to be brewing in October 1998 over whether mandatory inclusion of people with disabilities under 65 will occur for those who are Medicare eligible (Pear, 1998a).

Some insurers were ready to battle the government in court, but this action appeared to be unnecessary. A few weeks after the original report that suggested that HCFA would require that Medigap insurers underwrite care for people with disabilities who had lost coverage when their HMO withdrew coverage for Medicare beneficiaries, the insurance industry got the interpretation of the Balance Budget Act of 1997 that it was looking for. Administrator of HCFA, Nancy-Ann Min DeParle, ruled that "insurers did not have to start selling Medigap policies to disabled people under 65 if they had not done so in the past" (Pear, 1998b: A13).

Past procedures did not rule out access to Medigap insurance for people with disabilities. Sales to these individuals has been required by state law in 18 states. More legislation may increase that number in the future. With 30 states impacted by the notification by HMOs that they were pulling out of Medicare or reducing their service areas at the beginning of the new year, many of the current 444,000 affected enrollees, including people with disabilities, have become anxious about access to Medigap coverage and the extra expenditures that it entails. (State and federal regulation of managed care is discussed in more detail in chapter 9.)

The battle on the federal level may not be finished, even though the insurance industry is pleased with the current administrative ruling by HCFA. Consumer and disability advocates asserted in late 1998 that the Balance Budget Act of 1997 afforded protections for people with disabilities when their HMOs withdrew participation in the Medicare program. Once again, fear of financial risks, as found in pre-existing conditions that predict extensive utilization, dictate health insurance industry policy when profits are threatened.

FOLLOW-UP OF PEOPLE WITH DISABILITIES

The strategies, principles, and structural arrangements of managed care organizations, outlined earlier in this chapter, establish concerns among disability advocates and others who are concerned about the consequences of stinting on services for vulnerable populations. Starting in the 1970s, the planners of services in contemporary health care systems recognized that service substitution can involve regular or routine care outside of institutions. The tradition of care at home by a visiting nurse goes back even further in the twentieth century. Moreover, there is widespread agreement that being among family and familiar surroundings improves recovery from illness and enhances functioning for people with disabilities.

Home care has become part of the arsenal of care modalities in the late twentieth century, with this service being the fastest growing expenditure in Medicare. Vulnerability to cost containment could mean that home care, a substitute for admission to a skilled nursing facility following a hospital stay, might be limited in provider organizations with risk-based contracts. However, a team of nurse researchers, Adams, Kramer, and Wilson (1995), found similar quality outcomes when HMO home care patients were compared to fee-for-service patients.

Similar results were revealed when managed care programs for people with affective disorders were matched with fee-for-service psychiatric services. A British review article on studies in the United States did not find that cost containment meant lower quality of services for depressed elderly patients (Wells, 1995). Nor were patients' functional and well-being profiles along 12 domains different in three distinct programs self-selected by participants (Stewart et al., 1993).

These results may be reassuring when questions of quality of care are raised. However, most studies that compared outcomes between fee-for-service and HMO plans only followed patients for one year. Over a four-year period of observation, a sophisticated prospective investigation of 2,235 patients, conducted as part of the Medical Outcomes Study, found worse physical outcomes in HMOs than in the fee-for-service system (Ware et al., 1996). People with hypertension, non-insulin-dependent diabetes mellitus, recent acute myocardial infarction, congestive heart failure, and depressive disorders were followed from 1986 to 1990. Those chronically ill patients who were elderly and poor had worse physical health outcomes in HMOs than in fee-for-service plans. Patients with these characteristics were more than twice as likely to decline in health in an HMO than in a fee-for-service plan. Mental health outcomes were inconclusive and may be related to different HMO sites.

The demand for data on the impact of managed care on quality of services and health outcomes comes largely from the American Association of Health Plans, the trade association of managed care plans. Despite the risk of losing the battle to providers and regulators by having well-constructed outcome studies, the association has not retreated from its call for data on the quality of care. Even following the above-cited study by Ware and his associates that showed some morbidity and mortality results unfavorable to HMOs and other forms of managed care, these studies are needed to combat the reporting of anecdotes of medical neglect, even medical malpractice, through undertreatment. Still, there is no strategy for making this research tell a good story so that anecdotes do not have the only say in evaluating managed care. The popular press, the evening news, and even some home pages on the World Wide Web take the point of view that "if it bleeds it leads."

One Web site, "Fight Managed Care," contains 200 managed care horror stories collected from newspapers all over the country. Approximately one in five are about people with disabilities. In the first 25 horror stories, the contents of four newspaper reports related to disability are: denial of payment for supplies; wait-listing a child for six months for corrective surgery to determine if there was a surgeon in the plan who could perform the operation; and denial of payment for unapproved services received for treating seizures or multiple sclerosis.

These anecdotes in the mass media and their collectors are also followed up by the print and electronic journalists. Research results do not receive the same coverage. The current policy debate on how to correct managed care and the strong support in Congress for three different patient bill of rights legislation stem largely from these horror stories. The consumer protections this proposed legislation introduces is accompanied by provider protections as well. Some of the lobbying for legislation comes from specialty provider associations, whose members could be the big losers as the principles of managed care continue to support the view that "less is more." Consumers and providers alike want to regain lost ground in the backlash against cost containment as the driver of the system.

REFERENCES

Adams, C. E., Kramer, S., and Wilson, M. 1995. "Home health quality outcomes. Fee-for-service versus health maintenance organization enrollees." *Journal of Nursing Administration* 25 (11): 39–45.

Anderson, O. 1985. *Health Services in the United States.* Cambridge, MA: Ballinger.

Batavia, A. I. 1993. "Health care reform and people with disabilities." *Health Affairs* (Spring): 40–57.

Brooks, P. 1997. "Models of collaboration: Strategies for improving children's health in a managed care environment." In Ruth E. K. Stein, editor, *Health Care for Children: What's Right, What's Wrong, What's Next.* New York: United Hospital Fund.

Buchanan, J. L., et al. 1992. "HMOs for Medicaid: The road to financial independence is often poorly paved." *Journal of Health Politics, Policy and Law* 17 (Spring): 71–96.

Disability News Service. 1998. "Survey says: Disabled people's lot hasn't improved." *Disability News Service's E-News* 1 (August): 4–5.

Ebert, D. A., and Heckerling, P. S. 1998. "Communications disabilities among medical inpatients." *New England Journal of Medicine* 339 (July 23rd): 272–273.

Freund, D. A., and Lewit, E. M. 1993. "Managed care for children and pregnant women: Promises and pitfalls." *The Future of Children* 3 (Summer/Fall): 92–122.

Fuhrer, M. J. (editor). 1997. *Assessing Medical Rehabilitation Practices: The Promise of Outcomes Research.* Baltimore: Paul H. Brooks Publishing.

Gawande, A. 1998. "Medical dispatch: No mistake." *New Yorker* (March 30th): 74–81.

Gold, M., Nelson, L., Brown, R., Ciemnecki, A., Aizer, A., and Docteur, E. 1997. "Disabled Medicare beneficiaries in HMOs." *Health Affairs* 16 (September/October): 149–162.

Grembowski, D. E., Cook, K., Patrick, D. L., and Roussel, A. E. 1998. "Managed care and physician referral." *Medical Care Research and Review* 55 (March): 3–31.

Holahan, J., Coughlin, T., Ku, L., Lipson, D. J., and Rahan, S. 1995. "Insuring the poor through Section 1115 Medicaid Waivers." *Health Affairs* 14 (Spring): 199–216.

Iglehart, John K. 1994. "Health policy report: Physicians and the growth of managed care." *New England Journal of Medicine* 331: 1167–1171.

National Center for Health Statistics. 1987. *Family Out-of-Pocket Expenditures for Health Care, 1980.* National Medical Care Utilization and Expenditure Survey. Series B. Descriptive Report No. 11. DHHS pub., no. 8720211. Washington, DC: Public Health Service.

Pear, R. 1998a. "H.M.O.s cut off Medicare, leaving many in a quandary. Beneficiaries face new costs and policies." *New York Times* (October 19th): A10.

Pear, R. 1998b. "Government refines stand on Medicare and H.M.O.s." *New York Times* (October 24th): A13.

Stewart, A. L., Sherbourne, C. D., Wells, K. B., Burnam, M. A., Hays, R. D., and Ware, J. E., Jr. 1993. "Do depressed patients in different treatment settings have different levels of well-being and functioning?" *Journal of Consulting and Clinical Psychology* 61 (5): 849–857.

Ware, J. E., Bayliss, M. S., Rogers, W. H., Kosinski, M., and Tarlov, A. R. 1996. "Differences in 4-year health outcomes for elderly and poor, chronically ill patients treated in HMO and fee-for-service systems." *Journal of the American Medical Association* (October 2nd): 1039–1047.

Wells, K. B. 1995. "Cost containment and mental health outcomes: Experiences from US studies." *British Journal of Psychiatry—Supplement* 27 (April): 43–51.

West, J. A., Miller, N. H., Parker, K. M., Senneca, D., Ghandour, G., Clark, M., Greenwald, G., Heller, R. S., Fowler, M. B., and Debusk, R. F. 1997. "A comprehensive management system for heart failure improves clinical outcomes and reduces medical resource utilization." *The American Journal of Cardiology* 79: 58–63.

World Health Organization. 1998. *The International Classification of Impairments, Activities and Participation: Toward a Common Language for Functioning and Disablement. ICIDH-2.* Geneva: World Health Organization.

5

Contested Terrain: Access to Specialists and Hospital Stays

By 1997, the managed care revolution had caught up to most physicians in private practice. The Kaiser Family Foundation reported that 92 percent of physicians in practice had at least one managed care contract. The doctors surveyed also reported that 44 percent of their revenues came from managed care (Stolberg, 1998: A14). For many physicians, aside from an impact on their incomes, their control over their practices changed. Their once-seen-as loyal patients deserted them when their primary care providers did not participate in the managed care plans their employers provided. In many ways, physicians could not protect the values that made their work worthwhile to them.

In a series of articles, under the title, "After the Revolution," that appeared in a major national newspaper, journalist Sheryl Gay Stolberg followed the fallout for a single pediatric practice in a small idyllic town in northern California. Identifying a developmental disability is a complex process, often completed by a multidisciplinary team of professionals. In Placerville, a diagnosis of attention deficit disorder, not an easy one to make for a generalist, required a great deal of professional time. One doctor regretted that managed care would require that he see more patients in the course of a day to generate the same revenues he did before the heavy discounting required by MCOs. He would not be able to do as easily what he did that day—devote an hour to patiently question a high school boy to make a differential diagnosis.

Fast forward to the logic of cost containment in health care. Managed care organizations (MCOs) pride themselves on providing preventive care (e.g., immunizations, smoking cessation programs) and early detection measures (e.g., Pap smears, glaucoma testing) to their enrollees. Not only are these regarded as health protection measures, but they are inexpensive to conduct when compared to the tertiary care treatment involved in responding to such diseases as ovarian cancer, glaucoma, or emphysema. These forms of preventive care and early detection measures are strong selling points to benefits officers from large corporations and other decision makers who contract with an MCO. What do people with disabilities get in the way of early interventions in MCOs?

Advocates for the disabled argue that a health status screener and assessment for people with disabilities are important sources of information for practitioners. Whether a person with a disability enrolled in an MCO organization seeks treatment or not, it is useful to be prepared for the time when he or she will seek help. A baseline measure of health status allows the provider and the consumer to measure changes in health status over time. It also is a way of identifying problems that could use some new ways of working with the patient.

A health assessment asks the patient to rate current health status, make comparisons with one year past, and identify specific conditions for which he or she is receiving treatment. Additional questions concern household arrangements. Sources of social support, both inside and outside the household, are part of the assessment, as well as a complete history of current and past health care utilization, that is, from what sources and with what frequency.

These assessments are used in HMOs to screen a large population of publicly funded individuals who might tax an existing medical system. By surveying Medicare and Medicaid enrollees, an MCO can determine what kinds of support services it will have to establish and how much it will cost. Demographic information suggests this patient stream is going to be a burden and HMOs quickly act to organize their care.

Individuals with disabilities who enroll in an MCO through employer-based health care insurance, or some other kind of funding, are not subject to screening. In fact, although based on limited samples, my experience with Bob Griss (1998) of the Center on Disability and Health interviewing providers and managers in a midwestern city in 1997 found that even the total number of persons with disabilities in the MCO was an unknown fact. Since many disabilities are not visible or are disguised by those that bear them because of their stigmatizing quality, it is necessary to screen enrollees in order to provide quality care. With knowledge about patients' identities, however, providers get new responsibilities.

Estimates as to the number of enrollees with disabilities remains guesswork at MCOs, despite the presence of sophisticated information systems, the use of the International Classification of Disease-9 methodology, and a commitment to doing outcomes research. These data would be of great use in determining whether a procedure or intervention worked and for whom. Moreover, when there are data that refine diagnoses and determine if appropriate treatment has taken place, then providers have a better idea of what works in the prevention of secondary disabilities for people with disabilities. By treating these conditions or catching them early, resources can be preserved. In a highly integrated system, it is possible for care coordination or case management to target exactly what works for a person with a disability, just as they now are able to keep children up-to-date with their immunizations or regularly scheduled visits to the pediatrician. At this writing, there are few studies based on systematically collected data of how different kinds of approaches produce better or worse outcomes for people with disabilities. Evidence-based medicine, a promising area of research, does not exist in the area of health care for the disabled.

Despite the fact that there are few people with disabilities enrolled in MCOs, there is some evidence to suggest that those who now are enrolled, and even new enrollees, will, over the course of some years, "age on-site," and will become disabled. In the 1990s, access to health care is a problem that will not go away. For the news media, it remains the issue of the decade. Even conservative newspapers that fear more government regulation concede that there is much complaint evident among rank-and-file members of MCOs. While government regulation may be anathema, regulation in the service of the consumer is still supported widely by the American public.

What happens when people with expensive health care needs join HMOs? The managed care revolution has produced some positive results for Medicare-eligible people in rural areas, although the costs to the HMO led to its leaving that sector of Ohio in 1998 (Kilborn, 1998). This story is an extraordinary look at low- and moderate-income people, who often avoid getting all the care they need because some of it will have to be paid out-of-pocket. The base Medicare rate in rural areas did not match what was spent on Medicare subscribers in urban areas. The HMO folded its tent and abandoned many people who felt for the first time that the quality of their lives had made a definite improvement.

Many felt that the benefits available through the HMO were too good to be true. One 58-year-old woman, a diabetic who was also disabled following an accident at work, now could get many of the supplies and services she needed. This included eyeglasses, hearing aids, and dental care. Most important, she could get strips to test her blood sugar eight times a day. (A box of 50 strips costs $48.) Without the HMO, because of the high price of the strips, she was down to testing only four or five times a week.

Regular Medicare Part B required extensive co-payments for care or did not cover supplies. Many of those eligible did not acquire what has become known as "gap insurance" to cover many of the outpatient services, durable medical equipment, and supplies that they needed because of their chronic conditions. Some gave up these policies when they joined the HMO and now are having a difficult time getting gap insurance. There may be many thousands of other people with disabilities who have insurance that does not cover many of the items and services that they need.

There is survey evidence, courtesy of the media, that shows that enrollees worry about whether HMOs or other plans will be there for them when they need them. In 1998 the *Wall Street Journal* and NBC News conducted a nationwide telephone interview of 2,006 adults over a three-day period. A sample was drawn from 520 randomly selected geographic points in the continental United States. Each region generated a sample in proportion to its population and households with listed or unlisted numbers had an equal chance of being included (*Wall Street Journal*, 1998: A12).

Health was a major concern of all the respondents in the survey, even those with no immediate disabilities. Half of the poll respondents said they took a prescription drug every day. More than one-third of those surveyed said they have a chronic or serious medical condition that will last for many years. Almost half said they were at least 15 pounds overweight (Dunham, 1998: A10).

Despite these early warning signs of health problems, over 25 percent of the respondents had switched from indemnity insurance to an HMO during the past five years. While three out of four of those sampled were satisfied with their health care, 40 percent said that the national conversion to managed care was making things worse than in the past while only 20 percent thought it was making things better. It is no wonder that pressures for a "patient bill of rights" were being felt in Congress prior to the 1998 congressional elections. In a country that hates government regulation, a sizeable plurality in the survey favored legislation to promote HMO reform (Hunt, 1998: A9).

Even in the heart of Republican Dixie, there was a belief expressed that something needs to be done to correct abuses in HMOs. The most complaining people interviewed in the *Wall Street Journal*/NBC News effort to get beyond fix-alternative answers were those who had serious health care needs. A particular sense of powerlessness was expressed by a mother of two children with disabilities who worried about access to care. HMOs "have you at their mercy," said this Georgia native (Duff, 1998: A14).

The experiences of people with developmental disabilities or their care givers, often family members, speak to the need for care coordination or case management. Consumers need to be able to breach the bureaucratically imposed barriers between medical necessity and physical or occupational rehabilitation services that are desired by people with disabilities. Those that receive these services claim they prevent further deterioration or secondary disabilities. Furthermore, there is some information available to suggest that primary care physicians can act as advocates for individuals with disabilities to get the services that are believed to be needed. Whether advocacy involves extending benefits such as physical therapy, or getting access to subspecialists, there is often a tension that exists between policies aimed at cost containment and what is considered to be in the best interest of patients with disabilities. Anecdotes describing poor care can also be matched by stories in which families or consumers make it clear what they want within the confines of managed care.

THE LIMITS OF MANAGED CARE EXPLAINED

Several years ago, I conducted a focus group interview with five mothers of offspring with developmental disabilities, with ages ranging from the mid-30s to under five. A focus group interview is an excellent way to find out about the challenges of enrolling special needs populations in HMOs. My purpose was to examine how parents of children with developmental disabilities choose health care plans and evaluate their experiences in them. Some of these parents of older individuals with developmental disabilities were long-term members of HMOs. I was especially interested in hearing their stories since they recounted multiple experiences with their managed care plans.

In this effort, I adapted the *focus-group interview technique* to the study of consumer experiences with health services. Used by social scientists and market researchers for 50 years (Merton and Kendall, 1944), focus-group researchers learn close-up about the way in which decisions and preferences develop. Questioning in focus groups follows a funnel approach, moving from the general to the specific. To maximize the investigators' sensitivity to the concerns of the participants, the "questions vary in response to the character and requirements of each individual or group exchange" (Goldman and McDonald, 1987: 10). This session produced some interesting findings concerning experiences with HMOs, particularly for parents of children who had reached their adult years.

There were two important findings from this group interview. First, half the questions were *anticipated* and did not have to be asked because the parents were concerned with the issues behind the questions as much as we were. This indicated that the questions were revealing something important in their lives. Second, self-advocacy was an important skill in gaining access to services that were covered by the contract with a staffed HMO but might not be directly available.

What follows are some excerpts from this focus-group interview. In response to a question concerning how one respondent became involved with the HMO, a mother suggests the importance of continuity:

> We were covered by this HMO before my children with disabilities were born. With J., I realized something was wrong with his eyes. The HMO pediatrician could not figure it out. I got a referral to a specialist at Beth Israel. The HMO paid. We found out J. had congenital glaucoma. Over the years, one thing the HMO was not able to do was to give me specialists. For orthopedics, there is nobody . . . for seizures, there is nobody. They are there for pediatrics. Anything that I need them to write up, I have to dictate. They themselves are not trained to deal with our children. I had a pediatrician for all these years. When J. got sick recently as an adult and had to go to an ICU, I had to lose my pediatrician. I am altogether lost now because I have an internist who has never dealt with the handicapped. You asked why we stay with this HMO. I still have a pediatrician treating my 35-year-old son. Even after I stopped working for the city I picked it up to keep contact with her. They also made a referral to the Hospital for Special Surgery and this HMO paid. I had to fight with them for each payment over a number of years, but they paid for the orthopedist and for the appliances.

Typically, the responses to questions showed great variability when specialists were requested by parents.

> Did you ever give the name of a specialist whom you wanted the child to be referred to?
>
> *Respondent 1*: We are limited to HMO doctors.
>
> *Respondent 2*: My doctor did not hesitate to recommend an outside specialist to me that they paid for.
>
> *Respondent 3*: They wouldn't pay for a pulmonologist if they had one on their list.

Did you ever have difficulty getting access to a needed service?

Respondent 4: The HMO centers used to have physical therapists around but they never had people trained to deal with children with developmental disabilities.

Respondent 5: In my case I wanted my son to get physical therapy at the HMO. I was told that he can't get physical therapy because he was born with the condition. But they would give someone who got hurt on the job PT. If HMO is the thing of the future, parents have to be taught how to advocate with the staff. They have to be advocates for their kids.

If people with disabilities are enrolled in large numbers in HMOs or other managed care plans, they may not only have to fight for perceived needed services, but these plans may also lose their competitive advantages. The selection process for HMOs and other managed care plans has excluded many individuals with serious chronic illnesses and disabilities for two reasons. First, fewer of them are in the work force and therefore cannot gain access to plans that are tied largely to contracts with employers. People in the work force tend to be younger and healthier than the rest of the population. Given these characteristics, they bring fewer complicated medical problems to service providers. Second, whether we are considering adults or children, where serious chronic illness or disability is concerned, there is a great reluctance on the part of patients or their guardians to change from providers who may not be part of the various managed care networks and plans that exist. What advice can a benefits officer at a corporation give to an employee whose family can share in the savings afforded by participation in an HMO but who will be forced to give up an ongoing relationship with a pediatric cardiologist who has been treating since birth a child with a congenital heart defect? Clearly, many families will stick with what they know rather than take a chance on the unknown. Still, even those families who select a policy that permits unrestricted access to doctors who receive fee-for-service payments may find themselves subject to managed care provisions such as prior authorization for surgical procedures if the insurance company will pay for the procedure. For many people today this argument is academic since their employers offer but one managed care plan and no menu of choices.

Many plans utilize disease management providers for people with serious chronic illnesses such as diabetes. These programs are designed to reduce ER visits and admissions, improve outcomes, and reduce costs. In the past, these programs tended to be based on patients with the same severity levels and levels of compliance, as well as similar educational backgrounds, ages, and psychosocial needs. The avatars of disease management are now seeking to broaden their services to include patients with variability in all of the above-mentioned factors.

DISEASE MANAGEMENT AND DISABILITY

There are few models of disease management available with regard to disability. The availability of new therapies for patients with multiple sclerosis (MS), a chronic neurological disorder that affects more than 300,000 Americans, has led to the development of disease management programs that seek to reduce costs and the secondary disabilities associated with the condition. The symptoms of multiple sclerosis include loss of balance, tremors, stiffness, partial or complete paralysis, and short-term memory loss, among others. They occur when myelin, the insulation that protects nerve fibers in the central nervous system, becomes inflamed and/or breaks down (*Healthcare Demand and Disease Management*, 1998).

In intensive care coordination organized by a specially trained nurse, practice guidelines for MS are followed. Patient education takes place that stresses the need for people with multiple sclerosis to take certain precautions to avoid infections, adhere to their medication schedules to limit or delay debilitating effects of the disease, and avoid risks of falls in the home or at work.

The motivation for these measures is not strictly to improve the quality of life of the person with MS. Advocates of the use of clinical practice guidelines are also acutely aware of the cost saving for care where the yearly cost is more than $15,000 per MS patient. The use of nurses is justified by the costs offset in preventing pressure sores, broken bones, and skin breakdowns.

LIMITING BENEFITS

A less visible kind of restriction is the reduction in benefits for particular categories of intervention. Spurred on by the growth of managed care, in a recent piece of reasoned opinion, three lawyers and a physician raised and sought to answer the question as to who should determine when health care is medically necessary (Rosenbaum et al., 1999). One of the examples they used in their article pointed to the arbitrary nature of decision making to authorize benefits in managed care plans. A child with severe cerebral palsy was denied access to

> prescribed physical therapy to prevent muscular atrophy and possibly allow the child to walk. On the basis of a single article in a medical journal, how-

ever, the insurer's medical director decided that intensive physical therapy can never speed development of such children. A federal appeals court found the decision to be without any rational basis and required that the insurer cover the physical therapy. (231)

Similarly, some emerging treatments, such as the administration of growth hormones to children for the prevention of extremely short stature—a definite social disadvantage in American society—has been disapproved by insurers, despite almost unanimous recommendations by a great cross-section of practicing endocrinologists (Finkelstein et al., 1998).

By 1997 some of the executives of MCOs realized that the extension of speech, occupational, or physical therapy benefits for children, beyond the yearly allotted visits, was probably a good policy to pursue to deal with unhappy consumers. These kinds of arrangements rarely make the media, nor are they monitored carefully to see if they have more appropriate outcomes than in cases where benefits were not extended. It would be interesting to determine if these therapies made a difference for families as far as: (1) avoidance of secondary disabilities; (2) parent perception of school performance; (3) actual school performance, including attendance; (4) possible reductions in the use of other services, particularly hospitalization, what is known as a "cost-offset effect"; and (5) general satisfaction with services received. Since managed care is concerned with outcomes, this kind of follow-up study would be very useful. Finally, there is rarely any information collected on the characteristics of families and children who request and receive extended benefits that go beyond the plan's limits.

The benefits available under public insurance for people with disabilities has been subject to threatened limitation in state Medicaid programs. In 1998 the three-judge panel of the U.S. Court of Appeals for the Second Circuit found that the state of Connecticut was permitted to limit coverage. In the DeSario ruling, Connecticut was allowed to deny payments for durable medical equipment regarded as needed by physicians. In addition, some treatments were also denied.

The ruling was the result of the Connecticut Medicaid agency establishing a pre-approved list for medical equipment. Any apparatus not on the list would not be paid for, even when doctors recommended its use. Updating of the list seldom took place. Even if the device was seen as life saving by physicians, such as a machine to clear fluid from airways, the court ruled that the state had the right to ration care. Not only were disability advocates up in arms over this decision, but the nationally syndicated columnist Bob Herbert (1998) took up the cause, seeking to get the Health Care Finance Administration to rule on it.

To keep the costs of health plans competitive, managed care organizations also have set limits on hospital stays for drug abuse, alcohol abuse, and psychiatric care. The movement to contain costs makes these kinds of care less available. It should be noted that the cutbacks on these benefits in indemnity policies preceded the shift to managed care. MCOs have accelerated this trend while also reducing access to out-patient psychotherapy by contracting benefits and seeking deep discounts from providers.

BEHAVIORAL HEALTH CARE

Behavioral health care is a term used to refer to a discrete organization of the delivery of mental health services that MCOs contract for with a provider organization. The emphasis is cost containment through intensive case management and capitated payment for the entire basket of services used. Because it is based on rationing of services, to accomplish this goal of cost containment, providers agree to do only what the behavioral health organization designates as medically necessary and at discounted rates.

Mental health services have been a particular target of rationing, despite evidence that mental health services represent only about 8 percent of all revenues spent on health care annually in the United States. Because the perception among benefits managers was that employees were abusing their mental health benefits, often in collusion with their mental health providers, managed mental health care was originally touted as a way to cut costs (Saeman, 1997). Two specific areas where utilization was disproportionately high, inpatient adult and adolescent psychiatric care, allowed attention to be drawn to this health care sector, providing a screen on which to project concerns about costs. These services become "the ripest target" for scrutiny because it often appeared that no care coordination was taking place (Anders, 1996). Moreover, scandals in the for-profit mental health services sector in the 1980s, particularly in Texas, revealed lengthy stays that were medically unnecessary, and fueled this effort to deny care (Iglehart, 1996).

Concern about costs was abetted by a cultural movement to "debunk" psychology, often considered by conservative public intellectuals and talk show hosts as a handmaiden of the welfare state. Many of those who denied the efficacy of psychotherapy now jumped on the bandwagon. Debates about whether psychotherapy "works" became popular and providing psychotropic drugs rather than therapy became a way to cut costs (Rothbaum et al., 1998). Concerns about quality and ethics fell by the wayside. Restricting access to mental health care helped to cut costs (Anders, 1996). Benefits (e.g., fewer days lost from work) produced by clinical mental health interventions were ignored. A joke circulating in New Jersey in 1997 sardonically stated that an accurate advertisement for managed care, including managed mental health care, would be "Congratulations! You have chosen the cheapest plan with the poorest benefits."

Professional opinion against restrictions on benefits was manifest *before* the invention of behavioral health management service provider organizations. Not only have psychiatrists regarded the intervention of managed care companies in determining whether payment of long-term hospitalization will continue or be discontinued as irrational as well as adversarial, but they have argued in their own journals that such interference is harmful for the patient's recovery.

> If the patient shows signs of improvement, the insurance reviewer may insist on discharge; if the patient is making no progress, the reviewer may still insist on discharge on the basis of the premise that the treatment is merely custodial. (Gabbard et al., 1991: 319)

Critics of managed care applications to psychiatric treatment offer anecdotal information that suggests that the reviewers were trained in Alice-in-Wonderland logic rather than in psychiatry. Gabbard and his associates (1991: 318–323) analyzed managed care recently from a psychodynamic perspective. In essence they assessed the clinical impact of managed care review. If doctors take an oath to do no harm perhaps managed care companies, built around the use of medical expertise, need to be sworn in as well. Ever vigilant, managed care reviewers have created uncertainty for the already vulnerable patient who was making progress—but not in a straight line. Following an analysis of the borderline personality, these clinicians suggest through detailed case material that there are serious consequences for patients who have difficulty processing this information; moreover, treatment team members have difficulties working with a patient when they know that treatment time is limited; and families of patients are impacted upon as well when given a different view of the need for treatment by the reviewer. In sum, expectations of closing opportunities can create a sense of panic.

Managed care in psychiatric treatment did not stem only from rising costs. There has always been some bias in medicine against psychiatry, but even medical doctors know that there are real diseases that affect mental states and make people dangerous to themselves or others, or create real suffering in people who cannot fully take care of themselves. Moreover, the families of people suffering from psychoses or schizophrenia deserve intervention and/or relief from their burden.

There are some valid studies that demonstrate the importance of outpatient psychiatric treatment. Summarized in the April 16, 1992, issue of *The New England Journal of Medicine* by Leon Eisenberg, these studies show how depression can lead to more days lost from work than such chronic conditions as hypertension, diabetes, advanced coronary artery disease, angina pectoris, arthritis, back problems, lung problems, and gastrointestinal disorders. Depressed patients, identified by a structured telephone diagnostic interview, were worse off than medical patients in 17 of 24 pairwise comparisons. In a second study, based on a community-derived sample, the number of days bedridden for a sample of 3,000 patients was 4.5 times greater among those with major depression than in asymptomatic persons. The risk in persons with minor depression was 1.5 times greater than that in asymptomatic persons.

In sum, these studies show that disability days do occur for people with psychiatric symptoms and they need appropriate treatment. Not only is this humane, but it also makes good economic sense to do this since this treatment can lead to substantial cost offsets by reducing the use of other medical and surgical care. Psychosocial care needs to be viewed as a serious benefit, not a frill. How can this be done? There are three basic principles to guide the construction of any behavioral health care program.

First, the behavioral health providers of direct care and the primary care provider need to communicate frequently and work in partnership rather than as adversaries. There have been some instances where providers were able to work cooperatively for the patient's best interest. In general, however, insurers suspect psychiatric treatment, whether for inpatient or outpatient care, as being less valuable than care for physical illness. This bias is adopted by some employers who want to save money on health insurance for employees and their families. Biased cost cutting may be counterproductive since there is evidence that counseling services for workers reduce days lost through sickness or absenteeism.

Second, the intervention should be proactive as well as dealing with immediate distress. One of the things that patients being treated for mental illness can learn is how to avoid stresses that trigger a serious collapse. It should not be assumed that the neglect of psychiatric illness means that sooner or later the problem will resolve itself. Untreated psychiatric illness does have its costs to society and significant others. There is always the possibility of the intrapsychic stress manifesting itself in the form of physical illness or suicidal behavior. Unfortunately, psychiatric assessments and treatments are not viewed as preventive interventions.

Finally, psychiatric treatment can be accountable to insurance carriers. Utilization review is the form of peer accountability that has been generated by the American Psychiatric Association (APA), assuring that necessary and appropriate care is delivered. The APA developed peer review services in the early 1970s to give insurers the option of providing psychiatric care, limited only by medical necessity. This system has enabled insurers to achieve saving through cost avoidance in other areas of medical care. Psychiatrists review each case, working within guidelines established by the APA's *Manual of Psychiatric Peer Review.* Documentation of savings has been demonstrated with the private insurers, Aetna and Mutual of Omaha, and with CHAMPUS, the insurance system operated by the federal government for dependents of military personnel.

With these three principles in mind, an appropriate benefits package can be created that includes psychiatric care that allows healing time for serious cases and cuts down on the negative consequences of the failure to treat.

APPEARANCE AND DISABILITY

While the definition of disability used throughout this work refers to limitations on activities of living, there still appears as a background to conceptualization of disability the idea of stigma. A person born with a craniofacial abnormality or one who suffered the loss of the external part of an ear might be perfectly capable of working but would be put at a decided disadvantage when it came to competing with others for jobs, in the dating game, or in finding a mate.

Reconstructive surgery encompasses all kinds of interventions, ranging from those that make a person with a facial deformity look more like everybody else to those that involve making a person look younger or more fit. While it seems justifiable to say that a health insurance plan should not have to pay for a face-lift, a nose bob, or a tummy tuck, should it be allowed to refuse to pay for the construction of ears on an individual born without them, plastic surgery to cover scarification for someone who has been in a fire, or repair for a child born with extremely wide-set eyes and a sunken nose?

In the last example, one could argue that craniofacial surgery is simply cosmetic. Plastic and reconstructive surgeons may keep their charges down when it comes to making children look more normal but they are then forced to look for more cosmetic cases to off-set their financial losses.

Today enrollees in MCOs who require plastic or reconstructive surgery often have to contest the decisions of plan administrators when they request payment authorization for the many expensive operations they may require to look more normal. Appeals are the normal part of gaining coverage. Even federal legislation has been sponsored in the Senate to require plans to pay for reconstructive surgery following radical mastectomies (Jeffrey, 1998). This is clearly one of the areas of care where consumers say "there ought to be a law!"

It is ironic that we call for protection from the very plans to which we voluntarily sign up. (Some of the humor that accompanied the sclerotic growth of Soviet institutions could be applied here.) In many instances employers only sponsor one plan and one size must fit all. This is the beginning of the great divide between enrollees and their plans. It is also a barrier that is hard to anticipate. Utilization review includes case-by-case scrutiny of whether a procedure is medically necessary, along with a determination of the appropriateness of recommended interventions. Reviews can occur concurrently, retrospectively to determine the quality of decision making, or prospectively to establish need. Also bundled as part of utilization review are second opinions for surgery and requirements for precertification of a physician's request to perform a procedure.

Physicians, particularly those in the field of rehabilitation, often want to make life more normal for the disabled by helping them better pass among the normal through disguises that involve bodily changes. Sometimes it simply means reducing the intrusiveness of the stigma on face-to-face interaction. Providers often agree with people with disabilities that something therapeutic needs to be done but the MCO says no. Since people with disabilities often have comorbidities, this process to contain costs (and, in good faith, to protect the patient against unnecessary procedures) becomes contested terrain.

MEDICARE POLICY REGARDING EXPERIMENTAL PROCEDURES

Sometimes the efforts to prevent expenditures without evidence that shows that an outcome is effective are initiated by the payer for services rather than the HMO or other managed care plan. This has particular impact on the capacity of people with emphysema to fully engage in the activities defined by the Americans with Disabilities Act as major life activities.

The innovative surgical lung-volume reduction procedure has helped a small but significant minority of sufferers from this debilitating disease to live more actively and free themselves from reliance on oxygen when performing even the most unstrenuous activities. Surprisingly, HMOs and other private insurers were willing to pay for this thoracic surgery without the benefit of a systematic study where eligible candidates for the operation were randomly distributed into experimental and control groups. Those in the control group would receive the current medications used to treat emphysema.

Medicare, in response to the high mortality rate that occurred when the lung-reduction procedure was widely undertaken by surgeons, would only cover surgery for 2,200 patients in a nationwide research study co-sponsored by the National Institutes of Health. What is of most concern for patients who wind up in the control group is that they may have to wait up to five years to receive the surgery, or, if they can afford it, pay for the operation themselves. For ethicists, the concern again is that rationing is being organized according to the affordability of the procedure to the individual candidate (Gentry, 1998: A1).

Medicare, as the payer for care for almost 40 million Americans, is increasingly scrutinized by a Congress that seeks to limit the burden of this program on the taxpayer. Moreover, most physicians would agree that paying for worthless procedures and unproven medical technologies is not a good policy in this age of cost cutting, or any age. Therefore, testing whether a procedure is effective and worth the expenditures is of prime importance.

The managed care organizations, it seems, are less insulated from public demands to gain access to specialists and procedures than the Health Care Finance Administration, the federal agency that manages Medicare and Medicaid. They cannot appear cold and heartless when it comes to denying enrollees a procedure that has demonstrated modest success in improving the daily functioning of recipients. Public opinion, or the perception of consumer disgust, can impose on policy makers, leading them to make accommodations rather than hear about their cold and heartless ways. Asking members to wait five years for the completion of clinical trials involves more quality assurance than HMOs are willing to undertake in a competitive marketplace.

REFERENCES

Anders, G. 1996. *Health against Wealth: HMOs and the Breakdown of Medical Trust.* New York: Houghton Mifflin.

Duff, C. 1998. "Americans tell government to stay out—except in case of health care." *Wall Street Journal* (June 25th): A9, A14.

Dunham, K. 1998. "Concerns for health cut across social boundaries." *Wall Street Journal* (June 25th): A10.

Eisenberg, L. 1992. "Treating depression and anxiety in primary care: Closing the gap between knowledge and practice." *New England Journal of Medicine* 326 (April 16, 1992): 1080–1083.

Finkelstein, B. S., Silvers, J. B., Marrero, U., Neuhauser, D., and Cuttler, L. 1998. "Insurance coverage, physician recommendations, and access to emerging treatments." *Journal of the American Medical Association* 279: 294–302.

Gabbard, G. O., Takahashi, T., Davidson, J., Bauman-Bork, M., and Ensroth, K. 1991. "A psychodynamic perspective on the clinical impact of insurance review." *American Journal of Psychiatry* 148 (3) (March): 318–323.

Gentry, C. 1998. "Why Medicare covers a new lung surgery for just a few patients." *Wall Street Journal* (June 29th): A1, A10.

Goldman, A. E., and McDonald, S. S. 1987. *The Group Depth Interview: Principles and Practice.* Englewood Cliffs, NJ: Prentice-Hall.

Griss, Bob. 1998. "Quality assurance for persons with disabilities in commercial managed care plans." Unpublished report. Washington, DC: Center on Disability and Health.

Healthcare Demand and Disease Management. 1998. "DM programs take advantage of new therapies to reduce costs, complications, for MS patients." *Healthcare Demand and Disease Management* 4 (July): 106–108.

Herbert, B. 1998. "Health care denied." *New York Times* (July 26th): WK 15.

Hunt, A. R. 1998. "Politicians risk voter backlash this autumn if they ignore call for action." *Wall Street Journal* (June 25th): A9, A12.

Iglehart, J. A. 1996. "Health policy report: Managed care and mental health." *New England Journal of Medicine* 334 (January 11th): 131–135.

Jeffrey, N. A. 1998. "Corrective or cosmetic? Plastic surgery stirs a debate." *Wall Street Journal* (June 25th): B1, B23.

Kilborn, P. T. 1998. "End of H.M.O. for the elderly brings dismay in rural Ohio." *New York Times* (July 31st): 1.

Merton, R. K., and Kendall, P. L. 1944. "The focused interview." *American Journal of Sociology* 6 (May): 541–557.

Rosenbaum, S., Frankford, D. M., Moore, B., and Borzi, P. 1999. "Sounding board: Who should determine when health care is medically necessary?" *New England Journal of Medicine* 340 (January 21st): 229–232.

Rothbaum, P. A., Bernstein, D. M., Haller, O., Phelps, R., and Kohout, J. 1998. "New Jersey psychologists' report on managed mental health care." *Professional Psychology: Research and Practice* 29: 37–42.

Saeman, H. 1997. "Wall Street, more than managed care, responsible for health care changes, former psychiatry president declares." *The National Psychologist* (September/October): 18, 20.

Stolberg, G. S. 1998. "As doctors trade shingle for marquee, cries of woe." *New York Times* (August 3rd): A1, A14.

Wall Street Journal. 1998. "How the poll was conducted." *Wall Street Journal* (June 25th): A12.

6

Disability, the Quality of Life, and the Quality of Managed Care

There are two intellectual trails leading to concern about the quality of managed care for people with disabilities. The first is self-generated by people with disabilities who have often felt like second-class citizens. The movement toward greater integration and inclusion of people with disabilities into the mainstream of American life followed the civil rights movement for the elimination of state-sponsored legal barriers for African Americans. In the little-noted Rehabilitation Act of 1973, Section 504 struck at policies of discrimination found in public and private organizations in America through the power of the purse:

> No otherwise handicapped individual in the United States, as defined in section 7(6), shall, solely by reason of his handicap, be excluded from participation in, be denied the benefits of, or be subjected to discrimination under any program or activity receiving Federal financial assistance. (as quoted in Scotch, 1984: 4)

Not only was nondiscrimination the desired policy of the legislation that became known as Public Law 93–112, but as an unintended consequence, quality of life moved to the forefront of concern among disability advocates. The goal of nondiscrimination was to make it possible for individuals with disabilities to find competitive employment, live independently, and enjoy benefits of community living in a manner similar to that of other citizens.

In the 1980s, spurred on by the relocation from large and isolated institutions of many individuals with developmental disabilities or psychiatric disorders into community living arrangements (e.g., assisted living, group homes, hostels, half-way houses), the concern about the quality of life moved on to the agenda of disability advocacy organizations. There was a concerted effort to make these programs accountable to the clients served.

What was required in evaluating these services was a new way of thinking about individuals with disabilities. This concept included an increased respect for people with disabilities. Observers recognized that stigma was conferred when individuals were perceived as something to be tinkered with (in the language of Erving Goffman, "serviceable objects"), or something to be processed rather than heard.

Language-in-use seemed to matter and advocates sought to find designations that conferred power and status on those who were seen as diminished in some way. No longer conceived of as patients or clients, people with disabilities were now seen as consumers, even customers, whose responses to services were important. Measurement tools were created to determine if consumers perceived that the services received were promoting a sense of well-being, a feeling of belonging, and the freedom to choose what was needed, as seen from the point of view of a person with a disability. Quality-of-life measures have been developed for general use with the elderly (Hawkins et al., 1994), specifically for people with epilepsy (Devinsky et al., 1995), and for people with developmental disabilities (Schalock, 1996). Clearly, there is a conceptual correspondence between these measures and the approach taken by the developers of the ICIDH-2 classification of impairments, activities, and participation, as briefly described in chapter 4.

Consumers with disabilities not only had the opportunity to express themselves, they also had to learn how to get the things they needed from the delivery system. Parallel to the development of measures of satisfaction, the American Coalition of Citizens with Disabilities (ACCD) created the concept of self-advocacy; it carried out several projects in the 1980s to advance this concept. The ACCD sponsored advocacy education for pupils in the 9th through 12th grades to teach teenagers with disabilities how to gain access to the various systems that they will need to use as adults to secure employment, housing, recreation, transportation, and social services (Birenbaum and Cohen, 1985: 39). Self-advocacy training has also been adapted for use with people with developmental disabilities.

On another track, surprisingly, quality measures for health care delivery systems have been around since the early part of the twentieth century. Quality assurance in health care, while hardly ignoring consumer satisfaction, has been based on measurement concepts that are much more total-system oriented.

Ernest Codman, a Boston surgeon, kept careful records of the immediate and long-term outcomes of surgical procedures conducted at Massachusetts General Hospital. He reported on these findings in "The Product of a Hospital," a 1914 journal article, and in other publications (Brennan and Berwick, 1996: 96). Codman certainly set the agenda for a variety of approaches that followed in the next 80 years.

For Codman, a true pioneer and visionary, I suspect, the definition of quality that comes out of the "continuous quality improvement" tradition—that it is the right thing done at the right time, and done well— would have met his approval. What follows is a discussion of quality assurance mechanisms used before the rapid rise of managed care, and those that have developed over the past 10 years, as well as gaps in assuring quality of care for people with disabilities.

Within the subdiscipline of health care policy analysis, there grew a movement to establish some objective standards for determining whether a medical intervention was useful. Termed the "cost utility approach," it combined mortality outcomes—whether an intervention was life saving—with quality-of-life measurements. From the continuous investigation conducted for over two decades at the University of California, San Diego, researchers developed a general health policy model (GHPM). This theoretical model of health status includes the following distinct components: "life expectancy (mortality), functioning and symptoms (morbidity), preferences for observed functional status (utility) and duration of stay in health states (prognosis)" (Kaplan, 1992: 64).

Most important, from the perspective of disability interventions, the GHPM attempts to rank the various health outcomes according to their relative importance. An outcome of an intervention is assessed according to a quality-of-well-being scale, making it possible to determine the number of quality-adjusted life years that would result from a given intervention and how much it might cost. This approach takes a long-term view of an intervention, rather than seeing it at a single point in time. It is also possible to fold into the mix the impact of side effects to determine how many quality years result from a procedure.

The GHPM gives the consumer a chance to see what is being bought through medical practice. The cost-utility of services can be rank ordered. If an extremely expensive procedure is to get a high rank, it has to show that

many well-years are gained from it. Thus, a heart transplant, a costly procedure, will show more benefits if performed on a younger person than on an
older person because more well-years will be gained by a person with more
potential years to live.

Alternatively, there is some attempt to help those who need help the
most in this system of social selection. A procedure that will make a sick
person function better, someone who is starting at a lower rung on the ladder of health, should be performed over a procedure that would make the
same degree of improvement to someone already starting higher up on the
ladder. In this sense, when rationing occurs on a microlevel, it can be justified in terms of helping those who need the most help. If applied in medical
situations, this philosophy would certainly be helpful to people with disabilities. The question of who shall benefit is not, however, determined by
disinterested members of the community.

QUALITY ASSURANCE IN MANAGED CARE

The purchasers of HMO products are generally the benefits officers for
large corporations or government agencies with many employees. Their
major concern is the cost of the plan when considering which plans to
choose for employees (Freudenheim, 1996: D5). Service to employees is
also an important consideration, but the quality of care has not been of
great concern to corporate decision makers when deliberating whether to
stay with a plan or enter into a contract with a new HMO or another kind
of managed care organization. Because so many health plans exist in metropolitan regions, producing keen competition, purchasers of these services
may leave after one or two years when they find a better price elsewhere.
Slowly, buyers of health plans have shown increasing concern about how
good these HMOs are in delivering services, particularly when it comes to
keeping people well.

Predictably, quality may make the difference in the decision making of
purchasers when cost is basically the same. This lesson has not been lost on
the sellers. Eve A. Kerr and her associates (1996) created a questionnaire to
find out what kind of quality assurance programs were implemented by
capitated physician groups and to determine whether they emphasized
monitoring of overuse compared with underuse and improvement of preventive services rather than chronic disease care. The setting was a large
network-model HMO in California, with 133 contracting physician groups.
Ninety-four groups responded, representing 2.9 million covered lives.

The longer the physician group was in existence, the higher the profit-
ability; and the more capitation penetrated their markets, the more likely

the emphasis on quality assurance. The group's quality assurance programs monitored procedures subject to overuse, such as Caesarean delivery and angioplasty rates, more than underuse such as childhood immunization and performance of retinal examinations for diabetics. More effort was found in identifying underuse of preventive services than in follow-up services for people with chronic diseases. Enrollees were sent reminders for preventive services but not as frequently for chronic disease follow-ups.

Preventive activities are generally cost-effective and, as I have argued earlier, offset later expenditures, but they cannot be equated with all of health care. As people age, they become subject to chronic diseases, most of which can be managed with appropriate follow-up. While it is surely more difficult to measure the quality of chronic disease care than immunization rates, the overall effort to do so remains low. With such a strong emphasis on certain measures focusing on prevention and early detection of disease, physician groups and other managed care delivery systems may concentrate their service delivery in these areas, neglecting other parts of health care. Organizational observers note wryly that "what gets measured gets done." To answer the critics of managed care, it may be useful to redefine the scope of quality assurance to include processes and outcomes that are difficult to measure.

Some movement has been made nationally in that direction. The American Association of Health Plans, the rapidly growing MCO trade association, has spawned a quasi-independent organization that has generated complex review and evaluation standards to certify local or regional HMOs. Named the National Committee on Quality Assurance (NCQA), this organization has become the major source of information about the quality of care in HMOs.

Many HMOs, however, have made in-house efforts to collect data on their physicians' performances. For advertising purposes, plans may also participate in other quality assurance and consumer satisfaction studies. These efforts take time away from other tasks and are essentially duplicative. Parenthetically, if health care reform was successful, one standardized instrument would have served to make sure that consumers and purchasers had information on which to make decisions.

The development of quality assurance instruments has evolved from congressional concern about Medicare. In the 1970s, the Health Care Finance Administration developed utilization review and established peer auditing to ensure good care for Medicare patients. In addition, in the same decade, a creation of the American Hospital Association, the Joint Commission of Accreditation of Hospitals, sought to make sure that the quality of care was monitored in hospitals, and when indicated, efforts were made to improve clinical performance.

Today, the intense competition among plans has resulted in voluntary national efforts to establish base line comparisons between health plans. NCQA has led the quest for establishing valid and reliable indicators of plan performance and health outcomes. The availability of measuring tools also promotes interest in creating "report cards" for HMOs, with greater interest in establishing quality benchmarks than in the past. The pressure is increasing to learn about how well a plan does in treating diseases such as diabetes or glaucoma.

These results are recognized as critical to success in the managed care industry. The executives who run HMOs are concerned about making profits but that is not all they care about. Good marketing, as well as good management, requires information about how well a health plan does and about what kinds of patients are served. If an HMO is going to make money, it has to attract and hold on to subscribers as well as efficiently use resources. Organizing a health plan in a particular locality is built on planning, information, and a generalized positive attitude toward the enterprise. Finding out whether one is getting good value involves analyzing the conditions under which care is delivered, the performance of interventions and preventive activities that are medically appropriate, and good results—as measured best in improvement in health or the performance of the activities of daily living.

A program of good quality generates good results. It is based on the most valid knowledge about what works and what does not. An up-to-date physician does not continue to prescribe medicines that have been demonstrated to be ineffective or dangerous. In other words, a high quality delivery system uses systematically collected information strategically to obtain the most desired health outcomes. The LDS Hospital in Salt Lake City, Utah, is among one of the most advanced users of medical informatics and uses a complex information system to protect patients against errors (Finkelstein, 1998).

For at LDS 5,000 interlinked microcomputers instantaneously capture medical data from 25 different clinical areas and feed it into electronic patient charts. An artificial-intelligence system then scans this "real time" data for potential medical missteps. The computers can override incorrect prescriptions and change intravenous drip rates; they automatically page nurses if they encounter anomalous lab results and determine when patients can be safely taken off ventilators. Electronically, they report public health threats to local officials. Physicians can log onto computers at every bedside and order tests and view x-rays and vital signs. (28)

I question whether this advanced medical informatics is found in most MCOs. Quality is often measured by what is most easily captured by reporting. It is still hard to advise buyers of health plans as to which doctors associated with which HMOs make early diagnoses, avoid errors, and choose the right treatment (*Consumer Reports*, 1998). Some advocates for patients, and especially for people with disabilities, are starting to publicly recognize plans that correct bad or ineffective practices through quality improvement initiatives. Bob Griss, the director of the Center on Health and Disability, has begun to identify exemplary efforts by plans to accommodate people with disabilities. He presents this honor roll at his public presentations around the nation.

Sometimes the least expensive path to good outcomes is as good as the most expensive. Although inexpensive medications to treat cardiac problems produced by the blockage of arteries have worked quite well, less is not always more. Some expensive drug therapies are superior to less expensive ones, and not all patients respond to inexpensive products. This knowledge is gained through carefully controlled studies and the accumulation of epidemiological data collected on populations over long time periods.

Not all knowledge comes from rigorously performed studies. Administrative data are also useful in determining if resources are used efficiently. Information collection has been traditionally part of the management style of nonprofit as well as for-profit HMOs. Their management information services divisions have always collected a great deal of administrative data on how efficiently their providers use resources or whether there are some primary care providers with disproportionately high turnover or complaint rates. These activities generally fall under the heading of *quality assessment*, defined by the Institute of Medicine (1990) as "the act of measuring quality of care, of detecting problems of quality, or of finding examples of good performance."

What is new and interesting is the extent to which data are used to reassure the public, government officials, and leaders in medicine that the use of managed care will not mean second-rate care for enrollees. Meeting the NCQA criterion, sometimes called in a self-congratulatory manner by its public information releases "the gold standard," represents an effort to remain free of regulation and to reassure a skeptical public that HMO medicine is as good as any medicine available. This is done in several tried and true ways, although there are limits to the measures they use.

Less common than quality assessment is the Institute of Medicine's own "gold standard" for review—*quality assurance*. This applies to activities beyond assessment, extending not only to identifying the problem but also to verification, isolation of what can be corrected, initiation of interventions or corrections, and continuous monitoring to ensure that identified problems no longer exist. Furthermore, it seeks to make sure that no unintended negative consequences have surfaced during the correction process.

To understand the elements of a program designed to assess and assure quality, we need to examine how HMOs are constructed. The most important premise is that managed care be built on selectivity. It makes sense to the HMO planners to establish a health plan with the best doctors available and retain them so that patients will get the best quality care possible. Good physicians will also need to receive the appropriate administrative and allied health care supports for them to function well. Patients will need access to these providers and information on how to use the plan. For those patients who do not speak English, it would be useful if there were translators available or if some of the providers who spoke foreign languages would deliver their services, for example, taking medical histories in the patient's language. Those in charge of reviewing the quality of care determine how one health plan performs in comparison with another, based on the structure of services in place.

Determining whether a plan meets these expectations is a matter of reviewing the credentials of the providers and selecting not only those who are licensed but also those who have kept up with their fields of specialization. Being "board-certified" means in medical parlance that physicians have voluntarily taken a comprehensive test established by the specialty organization to which they belong and have passed that test. This test usually combines written and oral questions. The organizations that promote these examinations are sometimes called "academies" or "colleges" to indicate that they are scholarly in nature and not just in business to protect the material interests of the profession. So, for example, there are the American Academy of Pediatrics and the American College of Surgeons. After board-certification, the physicians may become a fellow in one of these organizations, which signifies that they have accomplished something and that these additional abbreviations after the M.D. represent certification. Most boards also require periodic recertification. HMO managers who are putting together a physician network or filling positions in a staffed-model program call this "credentialing."

HMO managers take the task of credentialing very seriously because of the prior aspersions cast upon doctors who worked in HMOs and/or were paid a salary rather than received fee-for-service remuneration. Historically, the American Medical Association, state medical associations, and the leaders of many county medical societies were contemptuous of HMO doctors, considering them failures who could not survive in private practice and who needed the security of salaries. While keeping up with one's field is admirable, no hard evidence exists that board-certified physicians produce better outcomes than those without certification.

Today, some consumers and providers continue to be convinced of the superiority of the physician who works outside of the HMO system, although it is very hard to support the statement that HMO doctors are inferior to those who work outside health plans. Many doctors belong to several plans at once, which makes for all kinds of new relationships between colleagues who may never have met. Where once surgeons only received referrals from primary care doctors whom they knew, they now receive authorization forms for consultations from doctors whom they never even heard of and certainly never met. Therefore, the idea of credentialing, though a selling-point to recruit enrollees, also reassures providers that they can trust the referrals they get and the subspecialists to whom they refer.

Establishing that the appropriate structure is in place for health care delivery only means that the stage is set for good care. Measures of performance occur in the field as well. These measures consist of simple or detailed examinations of what are considered standardized kinds of activities that assure the prevention of disease (e.g., immunizations), or testing for the presence of disease on a regular basis (e.g., doing a Pap smear). In addition, there are ways of determining if good care is delivered when disease is present. Children, for example, often get middle ear infections (otitis media). There are standardized treatment procedures for this condition and a process measure that is used to evaluate pediatric practice is whether those procedures were followed once the conditions were identified. Clinical practice guidelines are becoming more and more important as resources become scarcer and as efficiency becomes a recognized value in health-care delivery.

Perhaps the best measure of quality is the result of an intervention. These so-called outcomes refer to making people well enough so they can resume their normal activities. When a child with an ear infection receives an antibiotic promptly and is able to return to school quickly, missing fewer days than a child who is not treated in the same fashion, this is an indication that the medical intervention works, or works better when done sooner than later. Outcomes are the most desirable measures of quality. They can be studied rigorously to determine which kinds of procedures work best, or which providers get the best results. In addition, medical outcomes studies can tell us which patients respond best to the same intervention.

Outcomes are the broad measures of health status we come to expect from public health sources (Donabedian, 1988). These measures include survival, longevity, functioning, and physical comfort, to name some of the more objective measures. Subjective measures (such as perceived well-being and consumer satisfaction) are used when objective measures are not available or take too long to determine (Starfield, 1992; Stewart and Ware, 1992).

There is no more graphic example of outcome measures than the death rates of patients who underwent heart surgery. Cardiac artery bypass graft (CABG) surgery has been reviewed very closely to determine whether some surgeons have greater success than others in keeping patients alive. These studies of mortality attempt to control for the degree of impairment of the patient so that fair comparisons are possible. Some surgeons, perhaps even the very best, attract the sickest cardiac patients for whom the prognosis could be very poor. Biostatisticians adjust the risk associated with each patient so that there is a kind of level playing ground on which thoracic surgeons can compete. They have also discovered that the more operations performed, the better the success rate, suggesting that in complex tasks repetition remains a definite advantage. Some of these studies have also led to the discovery that those surgeons with the greatest success rates (i.e., capacity to keep their patients alive) prepare the patient differently than those with lower rates of success.

In some states, Pennsylvania, for example, these investigations have set a limit on who can perform bypass surgery, or cardiac artery bypass grafting. With the closing of some operating rooms and the restricting of this type of surgery to the certified, the mortality rate has gone down in Pennsylvania. Similar outcomes were found in New York State, where the Department of Health essentially restricted access to operating rooms of surgeons with poor outcomes in CABG. Additionally, the sharing of knowledge about preparatory procedures among the remaining approved surgeons has also improved outcomes.

The quality assurance teams established by NCQA have attempted to do all three of these measures—structure, process, and outcome. Every HMO that volunteers for review must complete detailed forms to receive accreditation, identifying who and what they have available to deliver services. These health plans also are encouraged to cooperate in an additional data-gathering effort with an instrument called HEDIS—the Health Plan Employer Data and Information Set. Now in its third generation, this instrument consists of eight domains that seek to assess the quality of each plan. An earlier version of HEDIS rated 330 health plans and the current version is built on this experience, plus the suggestions from various interested parties. These domains are

- Effectiveness of Care
- Access/Availability of Care
- Satisfaction with the Experience of Care

- Health Plan Stability
- Use of Services
- Cost of Care
- Informed Health Care Choices
- Health Plan Descriptive Information

New items are being tested out currently to determine if they can be used on a large scale. A substantial number of these new items relate to the effectiveness of care domain and some are public health oriented. These items include screening for the sexually transmitted disease chlamydia, and determining the number of people in the plan who smoke and who have quit smoking. Other new items are related directly to followup of abnormal test results, patient compliance with treatment, or patient management both in and outside of hospitals when serious chronic disease is presented.

This approach has a number of flaws, mainly because of its focus on what is most easily measured. There are a number of biases in what is essentially a performance or process evaluation of managed care organizations. The developers of HEDIS readily admit that more of the reviews of effective care are based on the use of preventive interventions, for example, immunizations for children or the use of standardized tests that are performed on people at the age when certain diseases usually have their onset. Usually, medical experts strongly recommend this kind of testing (e.g., mammography).

In response to criticism that followed earlier versions of HEDIS, there is much more of an attempt now to determine whether proper procedures were followed in treating people with such serious and life-threatening diseases as congestive heart failure. While these diseases are chosen to some extent because there are large numbers of individuals who contract them, more strategic reasons are behind the choice. Some of these procedures hold for all individuals with this disease and others are seen as necessary when information suggests that the patient is deteriorating or at risk of decline if nothing further is done. Such measures are deliberately included because there is evidence that taking action at such times makes a difference in patient outcomes.

There is also a glaring absence of measures related to conditions that are rare or of low prevalence in the population. The basis of this conscious decision on the part of the originators of HEDIS is that low-prevalence conditions or diseases do not provide a sufficient number of cases to satisfy the so-called power requirements of statistical tests needed to determine if differences between plans are not due to chance. Serious chronic conditions (e.g., diabetes) that affect large numbers of people generate enough cases in each plan to make comparisons across plans possible and even comparisons among patients within plans. Alternatively, rare conditions such as cystic fibrosis, which affects one out every 10,000 Americans, do not appear in sufficient numbers, even in the rare plan with one million members in a given region, to make powerful comparisons possible.

Access to care is as important as the effectiveness of care, especially if a person has a serious chronic illness or disability. HEDIS attempts to deal with the frequent criticism of managed care that enrollees do not get the care they need. When HMOs rely on primary care providers to perform gatekeeping functions, patient dissatisfaction or disappointment expressed in not getting to see a specialist may be expressed. A measure on whether consumers feel they experienced delays in getting care or a referral to a specialist is currently being evaluated for inclusion in a future reporting set.

For people with a serious chronic illness or disability it is just as important that the primary care provider has some experience taking care of people with special needs. If all of the primary care providers in a plan are unable to determine if a person with spina bifida is deteriorating because they have little experience caring for this sector of the population, then easy access in the form of being able to get an appointment within a week after calling may not be meaningful. The process of credentialing should include a systematic effort to contract with and train at least some primary care physicians or midlevel practitioners to identify these warning signs for people with neurologic or orthopedic impairments. Of course, if a plan wishes to keep such enrollees out of the plan, they could make a deliberate effort to avoid hiring or contracting with such providers precisely because they might attract expensive and difficult consumers with multiple problems. The delivery of quality services to seriously chronically ill or disabled individuals, at this point in time in the evolution of HMOs, will not be rewarded. The conscientious HMO may only attract more expensive cases, without enrolling any more of the healthy population whose capitation could offset the cost of delivery of complex and frequent services to those more in need.

Plans need to provide data on disenrollment to HEDIS. Such information could help determine overall satisfaction rates for a particular HMO and also identify whether those with serious chronic illnesses or disabilities disenroll at a disproportionately higher rate than the healthy.

Such information should be made available to potential purchasers of the services of this plan and current or future enrollees as well. HEDIS does look at whether a plan informs members about how the plan works. While this is required reporting, the specifications of HEDIS 3.0 do not indicate that it will provide a "drill down" capacity, as is found on the Internet, for individuals with special health care needs. This capacity shows if any special features can help them learn how to use the plan more effectively. In other words, upon request, more information is available that is tailored to the special concerns and interests of those with ongoing health problems.

Descriptive information on how the plan selects physicians, what policies exist on pre-authorization of services, and how the plan monitors and manages care for serious illness is part of the final domain in HEDIS. This domain provides detailed information on the plan's structure, staffing, rules and management philosophy. Under the subject of care management, a required measure is the approach taken in managing serious cases. As is stated in HEDIS 3.0 (NCQA, 1996):

Case management is the process of identifying patients at risk for costly care and developing ways to deliver quality care to these individuals. Each plan has its own methods of deciding which cases require case management, and creating services or programs for ongoing disease management and education. (49)

Clearly, this is an important tool designed to help patients get better or adapt to chronic conditions. But is it not important to determine whether case management is done in a particular plan to improve patient functioning, thereby demonstrating the effectiveness of care, or to conserve costly resources? The two goals—effective care and resource management—are not mutually exclusive, and sometimes the two clash. Reporting on the conditions under which this happens in case management, or better expressed as care coordination, makes it possible to determine what specific services become involved in what can be termed "judgment call" decision making and which plans tend to experience more or fewer of these clashes. Given this track record, potential enrollees can be advised what fate is in store for them, and plans can be rated as to how well they perform when care is vitally required.

Case management can orchestrate a variety of interventions, not all of them strictly medical. Some plans may make available a wide range of rehabilitation therapies to assist a patient following a stroke. Other plans may be very restrictive and reduce the possibility of delivering effective care. If HMOs are to deliver better care than fee-for-service medicine, then case management becomes crucial to make sure that patients get what they need, regardless of cost.

Plans that seriously fall behind the middle of the pack of all the HMOs may raise important questions as to the management of these plans and even the quality of the medicine practiced. Distinctions more precise than this may be very hard to achieve without creating misinformation for the public and regulatory agencies (Epstein, 1995: 59).

In certain areas, HMOs can rightfully pride themselves on the fact that they have been shown to produce greater benefits than fee-for-service medicine. Ease of access to primary care should produce a definite advantage in achieving early diagnoses of some life-threatening diseases, yet little process or outcome differences were reported in one investigation. A comparative study of the quality of care for colorectal cancer conducted at the University of Texas Health Science Center found no differences between fee-for-service and HMO cases for the duration of symptoms before diagnosis and several other parameters related to diagnosis, including rates of survival. Other differences such as time from detection to treatment made no difference with regard to survival rates after adjusting for age and stage of diagnosis (Vernon et al., 1992).

Similar results were found in a one year study of 5,295 people with rheumatoid arthritis cared for in fee-for service and prepaid group practice settings (Yelin, Criswell, and Feigenbaum, 1996). For 11 years, the study team followed 341 people. On either an annual or long-term basis, the quality of health care appeared similar for patients seen in either setting, with no differences shown in the number of office visits, outpatient surgeries, hospital admissions, and painful joints.

While HEDIS 3.0 included a domain on satisfaction with the experience of care that should be sensitive to some of the access issues raised in the preceding discussion of case management, there were no specific questions addressed to consumers about how people with chronic illnesses or disabilities fare in HMOs. Fortunately, a national survey, the Consumer Assessment of Health Plans, is planning to include a substantial set of questions on what health plan enrollees with such conditions experience with regard to access to specialists and therapies. Comprised of six sections, this instrument does not limit itself to HMO members but will reach consumers with indemnity insurance or those who are covered by a preferred provider organization. The survey questions focus on the last medical visit and what was the consumer's experience during the last six months (Department of Health Policy, Harvard Medical School, 1996).

This survey seeks to gain information about utilization, access, and the degree of satisfaction with services. It also has a goal of determining whether various problems identified by consumers are attributed to health plans or providers. This means that gaining access to needed care or approval or referrals or pre-authorization by the plan is a central concern of the researchers. Some specific questions are:

- In the last six months, have you had any problems arranging to see a specialist who has adequate experience evaluating and treating a specific condition you have?

- In the last six months, has your health insurance plan refused to approve or pay for any medical care or tests that you thought you needed?

- In the last six months, have you postponed or gone without medical care or medicine that you needed because your health insurance didn't cover it?

It is possible to compare similar populations in fee-for-service and capitation plans to determine whether they have equal access to care. Mauldon and colleagues (1994) compared the extent to which children with special needs in a single HMO over a two-month period have comparable access to acute care visits and check-ups as those in the fee-for-service system. Few differences in use of the health services were found. However, given the fact that major disabling conditions were present in this sample of 1,685 children, it would have made for a more crucial comparison to see whether access to specialty care was similar or different. After all, few pediatric providers can manage on their own conditions such as blindness, diabetes, cerebral palsy, mental retardation, and amputations.

This raises another important consideration. In a highly cost-conscious service environment, some observers have suggested that there may be some reluctance to introduce new treatment modalities when they are either not part of the standard benefit package or are likely to increase expenses (Ireys, Grason, and Guyer, 1996). Similarly, lock-step protocols for providers do not always allow for the use of clinical judgment, especially when it costs the plan money (Herbert, 1996).

Concern about the quality of care in HMOs has also become the responsibility of the Health Care Financing Administration (HCFA), with almost 10 percent of Medicare beneficiaries in health plans, and 74 percent having access to at least one managed care plan. Enrollments were growing in 1995 at 75,000 a month and future efforts to reduce the cost of the Medicare program will be built on encouraging senior citizens to choose HMOs, leading to even greater recruitment. Former HCFA director Bruce Vladeck (1995) has indicated that more frequent on-site monitoring will occur at HMOs that enroll many Medicare beneficiaries. In addition, a greater effort will be made to educate enrollees concerning their appeal rights and the appeal process. While HMO members who are Medicaid beneficiaries need to know their rights, HCFA lost a court battle in October 1996 over whether a beneficiary loses the protections of HCFA when he or she enrolls in an HMO. A three-judge federal appeals court in California ruled in 1998 that Medicare patients were entitled to "due process" in the form of immediate hearings, legible notifications of denials of services and how to appeal those denials, and access to disclosure statements when denied care by HMOs (Pear, 1998). This is a significant validation of the lower court ruling and will require that HCFA enforce the rights of elderly and disabled people in Medicare HMOs.

HCFA is working to develop measures of quality for the Medicare population and is collaborating with HEDIS and the newly organized Foundation for Accountability (FACCT). Not a creature of the health plans, FACCT is the brain child of Dr. Paul Elwood, the father of managed competition, and some of the current major purchasers of managed care, representing 80 million covered lives. Both public purchasers such as the Federal Employees Health Benefits Program and private purchasers such as the General Motors Corporation are represented on the FACCT Board of Trustees. Representatives from major consumer groups also sit on the board, including those from the American Association of Retired Persons and the National Alliance for the Mentally Ill.

FACCT focuses on generating better information about the quality of health care by developing valid measures of the output of health care organizations, including consumer satisfaction, that can be disseminated to consumers throughout the United States. Founded in 1995, the following year this organization created five sets of quality measures focusing on breast cancer, diabetes, major depressive disorder, health risks, and health plan satisfaction.

An alliance of purchasers, consumers, and health policy experts focusing on accountability is promising. What they are attempting to measure is not related to the strong points of managed care but should shed light on the effectiveness of HMOs in handling difficult tasks. This kind of approach pays more attention to chronic illness than HEDIS or the Consumer Assessment of Health Plan Survey (CAHPS). The instrument is less burdensome to complete, and is aimed at universal application so the quality of care can be compared across all HMOs.

QUALITY MANAGEMENT IN HMOS

While these national efforts produce "report cards" on various HMOs, they are not designed to identify on a system-wide basis why problems exist in different HMOs and how they can be corrected. Independent of the quality assessment programs undertaken by NCQA is the movement toward continuous quality improvement, a spinoff of the work of the revered statistician W. E. Deming. This approach has been institutionalized in hospital management through the work of Berwick, Godfrey and Roessner (1990).

Following these leads, the large HMO, United HealthCare, created a continuous quality improvement program called Quality Screening and Management. Using HEDIS-collected claims data, analysts identify problems in the making. Then medical record analysis provides the data to validate performance that can be improved. Management interventions are designed to deal with these problems. Finally, a review takes place of the same records to determine whether improvements have been instigated. This kind of work holds a great deal of promise for improvements in all kinds of complex health systems, not just HMOs. In fact, it is a technique of quality improvement found in many different industries, commercial businesses, and even government.

LESSONS FROM MEDICAID MANDATORY MANAGED CARE PROGRAMS

When all Medicaid beneficiaries are required to receive their medical care from HMOs, there are few options for beneficiaries to go back to fee-for-service medicine. Several states that have mandatory managed care have recognized this problem and have made attempts to head off consumer dissatisfaction by bringing Medicaid-eligible individuals into the planning process. Note that here the intellectual trails adumbrated at the beginning of this chapter merge: the idea of self-advocacy along with consumer satisfaction approaches melds into the quality assurance tradition. Hopefully, this process will generate a more sensitive health care system.

In Oregon, for example, disability advocates felt they would not gain access to specialty care because of HMO rules and regulations. Consensus building was a goal of the program planners in Oregon (United States General Accounting Office, 1996):

> For more than a year before bringing disabled beneficiaries into managed care, Oregon's Medicaid staff held weekly meetings with health plan representatives, beneficiary representatives, and state social service agencies (from whom most disabled residents received case management services). (36)

Discussions in Arizona as well as Oregon dealt with building common definitions of such terms as case management, "medical necessity," habilitation, and disability. Arriving at acceptable definitions of these terms is very important to the disability community where often care that maintains functioning and prevents deterioration is denied because no improvements can be expected.

In three states with mandatory Medicaid managed care there were ongoing meetings between the interested parties after conversion to capitation. Beyond achieving consensus, Medicaid officials worked with the medical directors of the various health plans to develop clinical practice guidelines and procedures for evaluating new treatments and technologies.

Aside from the benefits of case management or care coordination, the methods of quality assurance need to be able to look closely at the outcomes due to provider intervention, holding constant the various environmental influences that can make for better or worse results. Furthermore, to focus on provider intervention, better measures of risk need to be developed so that providers who have a disproportionately high-risk patient panel with a specific serious chronic illness or disability will not be compared to their peers with a different case mix. Because risk-adjustment is so difficult, HEDIS has not included it in its methodology.

When HMOs fail to develop a case management model or have no concept of interdisciplinary teams to deal with serious chronic illness and disability, then state departments of health need to make plans accountable. One way they can do that is to insist that approval of HMOs is contingent on contracts with specialty care centers, sometimes called "centers of excellence," where access to services is not prejudiced by organizational cultures that value limiting expenditures over quality care. It is almost as if health plans have to be protected against their better features of rationing to keep them from denying access to specialty services for those who appropriately need them. Health plans have to learn about specialty care centers, why they are useful, and how to work cooperatively with them.

Finally, for measures of quality to be truly valid, there needs to be "sensitivity to changes induced by conservation of resources" (Epstein, 1996: 227). Plans that use fewer resources may be placing their enrollees at risk while realizing savings in costs. Consumers need to be protected against decisions made to control providers because of the global budgeting produced by a prospective capitation payment system. When we are patients we may not have sufficient knowledge or expertise to recognize the dangers of conservation, just as we often do not recognize the dangers of overtreatment in fee-for-service medicine and indemnity insurance.

REFERENCES

Berwick, D. M., Godfrey, A. B., and Roessner, J. 1990. *Curing Health Care: New Strategies for Quality Improvement.* San Francisco: Jossey-Bass Publishers.

Birenbaum, A., and Cohen, H. J. 1985. *Community Services for the Mentally Retarded.* Totowa, NJ: Rowman & Allanheld.

Brennan, T. A., and Berwick, D. M. 1996. *New Rules: Regulation, Markets, and the Quality of American Health Care*. San Francisco: Jossey-Bass.

Consumer Reports. 1998. "In search of quality health care: Access and price have dominated the health-care debate. Few are talking about quality." *Consumer Reports* (October): 35–40.

Department of Health Care Policy. 1996. "Consumer assessment of health plans. Chronic condition version." Unpublished paper. Cambridge, MA: Harvard Medical School.

Devinsky, O., Vickney, B. G., Cramer, J. A., Perrine, K., Hermann, B., Meador, K., and Hays, R. D. 1995. "Development of the quality of life in epilepsy inventory." *Epilepsia* 36: 1089–1104.

Donabedian, A. 1988. "The quality of care: How can it be assessed?" *Journal of the American Medical Association* 250 (12): 1743–1748.

Epstein, A. 1996. "The role of quality measurement in a competitive marketplace." In S. H. Altman and U. E. Reinhardt, editors, *Strategic Choices for a Changing Health Care System*. Chicago: Health Care Administration Press.

Epstein, A. 1995. "Performance reports on quality—Prototypes, problems and prospects." *New England Journal of Medicine* 333 (July 6th): 57–61.

Finkelstein, K. E. 1998. "The computer cure." *The New Republic* (September 14th and 21st): 28–33.

Freudenheim, M. 1996. "The grading becomes stricter on H.M.O.s." *New York Times* (July 16th): D1, D5.

Hawkins, B. A., Eklund, S. J., Kim, K., and Greene, K. 1994. *Five Dimensional Life Satisfaction Index*. Bloomington: Indiana University, Center on Aging and Aged.

Herbert, B. 1996. "In America: Mugged in the hospital." *New York Times* (August 8th): A27.

Institute of Medicine. 1990. *Medicare: A Strategy for Quality Assurance* (Vols. 1 and 2). Washington, DC: National Academy Press.

Ireys, H. T., Grason, H. A., and Guyer, B. 1996. "Assuring quality of care for children with special needs in managed care organizations: Roles for pediatricians." *Pediatrics* 98 (2): 178–185.

Kaplan, R. 1992. In M. A. Strosberg, J. M. Wiener, and R. Baker, with I. A. Fein, editors, *Rationing America's Medical Care: The Oregon Plan and Beyond*. Washington, DC: The Brookings Institution.

Kerr, E. A., Mittman, B. S., Hays, R. D., Leake, B., and Brook, R. H. 1996. "Quality assurance in capitated physician groups: Where is the emphasis?" *Journal of the American Medical Association* 276 (October 16th): 1236–1239.

Leatherman, S., Peterson, E., Heinen, L., and Quam, L. 1991. "Quality screening and management using claims data in a managed care setting." *Quality Review Bulletin* 17 (11): 349–359.

Mauldon, J., Leibowitz, A., Buchanan, J. L., Danberg, C., and McGuigan, K. A. 1994. "Rationing or rationalizing children's medical care: Comparison of Medicaid HMO with fee-for-service care." *American Journal of Public Health* 84: 899–904.

National Committee on Quality Assurance (NCQA). 1996. "HEDIS 3.0 draft." Unpublished paper. Washington, DC: NCQA.

Pear, R. 1998. "Court backs protections for Medicare patients denied by H.M.O.s." *New York Times* (August 14th). http://www.nytimes.com/y. . . pol/healthcare-suit.html

Schalock, R. L. (Ed.). 1996. *Quality of Life. Volume I: Conceptualization and Measurement.* Washington, DC: American Association on Mental Retardation.

Scotch, R. K. 1984. *From Good Will to Civil Rights: Transforming Federal Disability Policy.* Philadelphia: Temple University Press.

Starfield, B. 1992. *Primary Care: Concept, Evaluation and Policy.* New York: Oxford University Press.

Stewart, A. L., and Ware, J. E., Jr. 1992. *Measuring Functioning and Well-Being: The Medical Outcomes Study Approach.* Durham, NC: Duke University Press.

United States General Accounting Office. 1996. *Medicaid Managed Care: Serving the Disabled Challenges State Programs* (pp. 96–136). Washington, DC: GAO/HHS.

Vernon, S. W., Hughes, J. I., Heckel, V. M., and Jackson, G. L. 1990. "Quality of care for colorectal cancer in a fee-for-service and health maintenance organization practice." *Cancer* 69 (10): 2418–2425.

Vladeck, B. C. 1995. "Statement before the Special Committee on Aging, U.S. Senate." August 3rd. http://www.hcfa.gov/testimony/t080395.html

Yelin, E. H., Criswell, L. A., and Feigenbaum, P. G. 1996. "Health care utilization and outcomes among persons with rheumatoid arthritis in fee-for-service and prepaid group practice settings." *Journal of the American Medical Association* 276 (October 2nd): 1048–1053.

7

Managed Care and Centers of Excellence

The original Clinton Health Security Act called for a partnership between managed care organizations and what were designated as "centers of excellence." This expression referred to, in general, academic medical centers (locations for tertiary care), even specialized diagnostic and evaluation units (e.g., for developmental disabilities) that were usually found in academic medical centers, or, similarly situated, treatment centers for rare and sometimes costly conditions (e.g., hemophilia). What the health care reform task force planners tried to do was to manage competition so that these institutions would not be eliminated in a "race to the bottom" to deliver services at the lowest price. In the vision of the planners, MCOs were to seek services from these existing citadels rather than reconstruct them. Interestingly, the health care reform task force that was assembled by Hillary Rodham Clinton did not include much representation from the medical schools of the United States.

With the defeat of serious health care reform in 1994, the well-capitalized growth of managed care has accelerated. Under managed care, the integration of services and restricted access to hospitals and specialty care has created fewer options for the directors of these centers of excellence. From their point of view, at best, managed care is not necessarily the enemy. However, few of these leaders would argue that it is their friend. If left on its own, its revolutionary impact on financing and organization will destroy much that is good as well as rein in the cost of health care. It needs to be made to accommodate the complex functions of academic medical centers (AMC)—long known to deliver care to the uninsured, conduct clinical research, and train physicians.

The growth of managed care has been deemed the reason why the current rate of inflation in health care costs is well below the high rates of the 1980s. While the rate of cost growth may be diminishing, the problem of access for those without insurance remains. The greater efficiency in health care delivery introduced by HMOs has not done much to extend coverage to the uninsured, except in states that reformed their Medicaid system to include more of the uninsured (Oregon, Tennessee). Nor has managed care been regarded by consumers as producing better care at less cost. As mentioned earlier, studies that measure consumer satisfaction with health plans, while demonstrating satisfaction within the same range as levels for fee-for-service plans, often reflect respondents' concerns about whether the plan will be there for them if they have complex medical problems.

Centers of excellence earn their reputations as tertiary care centers that deal with the most complex medical problems. AMCs are, at the same time, multifunctional institutions. Many of the tasks of medicine involve the continuous rebuilding of its infrastructure through the creation of new knowledge and the renewal of the human capital through having trainees or residents deal with the most difficult cases. In addition, these practical citadels of twentieth-century health care have been often the sources of charity care for those without insurance, including the homeless, undocumented aliens, or the near-poor who cannot qualify for Medicaid, with the funding coming largely from indemnity insurance payments that generated a surplus for these nonprofit corporations. These important functions in our health care system are weakened by the penetration of markets by managed care organizations and their consequent reduction in referrals and demands for lower fees.

Today, as part of AMCs, hospitals are becoming more and more dependent on contracts with HMOs for inpatient care. Consequently, there will be fewer resources in their budgets to provide charity care for the uninsured. To their credit, hospitals and medical centers delivered uncompensated care through surpluses derived from the per diem payments generated by third-party and out-of-pocket payers. Even with the shift in the last decade to a prospective payment system for Medicare patients and subsequently for those with commercial insurance, there was an attempt to provide emergency care as well as hospital care for individuals without insurance. Congress also prevented hospitals receiving federal assistance from turning away patients who had no insurance and could not afford to pay for services from emergency departments. Moreover, hospitals that had a disproportionate share of the burden of caring for the poor, the uninsured, and the elderly also received subsidies through legislative funding provisions for Medicare and Medicaid.

The reduction in revenues for medical care impacts also on other functions. Clinical research in AMCs has been built partly on the capacity of scientists who were also medical doctors to have access to mechanisms to fund some research activities with clinical revenues. In the days when costs were not seen as a major concern, research projects could be initiated and conducted in a manner so that the actual equipment and labor time were buried in per diem costs. The comfortable relationship between payers and providers meant that some procedures performed on patients or specimens taken from them helped advance knowledge rather than benefiting directly the patient being treated. Today, some patient care services provided in hospitals may be regarded by HMOs as research related and therefore not activities that represent valid charges related to a hospital stay.

Now, with fees-for-service being deeply discounted, the specialist who is based in the AMC often has to spend five or more days to generate the amount of income that previously came from four days of consultations. Time for research is less available than it once was. With the arrival of HMOs on the scene, the old assumptions no longer hold when it comes to sustaining clinical research. A new arrangement, perhaps a new partnership, needs to be created. However, it will take some time to create this new compact.

Just as there is now fear that research will suffer with this new payment mechanism and system of organizing medical work, there is also concern that medical training will suffer. Traditionally, attending physicians devoted a portion of their day on site at hospitals and medical centers to teaching house staff (interns and residents) and/or medical students about some of the aspects of care and how to deal with patients. Now with primary-care physicians (PCPs) working under a capitation mechanism, there is far less control over one's schedule than in the past. In HMOs, with high PCP-to-patient ratios, there is little flexibility in the working day so there is little time to devote to teaching the next generation of physicians some of the finer points of care.

Specialists face a similar problem, although they may not be expected by contract to see as many patients per day. Again, the deep discounts from the standard fee that HMOs demand from participating physicians, in exchange for large numbers of referrals, means that doctors need to do more to reach the same level of remuneration than they did before the advent of managed care. While teaching in AMCs was often donated or pro bono labor in the past, it was a valued and esteemed activity. There are serious concerns at these centers as to how to make up for the shortfall in mentoring that once was assumed to come with the territory when a doctor received admitting privileges to a hospital.

The support of these activities was part of the "connective tissue" that held American society together. Plans for reforming health care, while grand in scope, always recognized these important functions of AMCs. While never perfect, these institutions and their efforts to survive through mergers are barometers today of a new health care crisis. Quality, access, and cost—the trinity of problems that made single payer an option and created the Clintons' Health Security Act—are back on the national agenda. Current legislative proposals seek to make sure that quality and access are not eclipsed by cost considerations.

Funding for AMCs could come from a tax on health insurance or managed care organizations. Distribution of funds should take into account the overproduction of specialists from these programs and create incentives to limit their numbers. We need to make sure that our world class medical care and concomitant research and training programs are available for all Americans—embedded in all delivery systems—and are not just a memory.

NEW FORMS OF MEDICAL ORGANIZATION AND CENTERS OF EXCELLENCE

The reorganization of health care financing through managed care calls into question the capacity of specialty services to maintain quality of care and ease of consumer access, given the new demands of tightly knit delivery systems. Integrated Provider Associations (IPAs) are medical center/physician networks established in a particular region. They often become the delivery systems for a number of privately and publicly financed managed care organizations.

IPA leadership must make important decisions in the creation of a "full-service" system. Working with limited premium dollars, an IPA has to make precise distributions of resources, because under these new systems of financing, cross-subsidization will be less and less possible. Thus, to make the product they sell to MCOs competitively priced, IPAs often extract discounts from practitioners and seek other less costly solutions to medical care problems.

IPA decision makers must determine if existing centers of excellence are affordable under these new constraints. Leaders must decide whether to invite into the IPA not only primary care providers (PCPs) but also highly specialized units at academic medical centers (AMCs), such as centers of excellence. These decisions are somewhat different from allowing "any willing provider" to participate in a network, or the subsequent step of credentialing PCPs, because of the complexity of the units being considered for integration into the IPA.

Through the use of a multidisciplinary approach, some programs that deliver specialized services to people with serious chronic illnesses and/or disabilities have developed high quality services. They have evolved from specialty clinics held one day a week at a local hospital, where patients with a particular disease were seen by a few interested medical specialists, to major specialty centers drawing patients from a wide radius. These centers are currently financed mainly by third-party payments from private or public insurers; special government subsidies and training grants also help to offset the high costs of multidisciplinary diagnostic and therapeutic services as well as clinical teaching.

Health policy analysts need to study the following questions: Under what conditions should IPA leaders utilize the services, such as diagnoses, evaluations, and therapies, required by patients with serious chronic illness and/or disabilities, that individual providers or existing regional centers of excellence offer? Also, given the complexity of these patients' needs, and the low prevalence of many of these conditions, which providers, nurses, PCPs, or specialists should become the case managers/coordinators of this care? To what extent are care coordination skills transferable from dealing with one type of disease to another, or, alternatively, to be effective, must case managers develop skills related to specific groups of diseases, e.g., neurologic disorders?

Additionally, how is medical training affected by decisions to follow the least expensive pathway to service delivery? To what extent will specialty programs have the opportunity to inform future or newly practicing physicians about the services they provide and why a multidisciplinary team approach is productive for patients? Finally, is there public awareness and involvement in decisions about services that impact on the quality of life of people with serious chronic diseases and/or disabilities?

To answer these questions, we need to examine how current changes in the financing and vertical and horizontal integration of health care affect the provision of coordinated and comprehensive diagnostic and therapeutic services for special needs populations that were previously found only in centers of excellence. This objective could be accomplished through a synthesis of knowledge about how IPAs conceive of these services, deliver them either through collaboration with centers of excellence, or by some other means.

The New York City Metropolitan Region, for example, is an excellent setting to study the consequences of integration of the health care system. Data on individual practitioners indicate that many belong to more than five managed care plans. By 1997, according to the Greater New York Hospital Association, 112 out of 125 area hospitals were part of nine multihospital systems. The modal type was a five to nine hospital system, containing over half the multihospital systems in the region.

Given this trend toward integration, 85 percent of the systems in the region sponsor a physician organization. Yet many of the system-affiliated physicians remain outside of these physician organizations, perhaps because they are salaried employees of AMCs or other health care delivery organizations. We need to look at the consequences for future care of these organizational developments at AMCs: How do they and their units respond to the changing health care environment? Are professional activities continued when referrals decrease and/or funding of graduate medical education via Medicare allocations is reduced sharply? Who negotiates for them with the newly formed health systems? What happens when centers of excellence become redefined from being "profit centers" to being "cost centers" because payers are reassigning risk to providers?

Additional data gathering should take place in metropolitan regions such as Miami, Minneapolis/St. Paul, and the San Francisco Bay area, where managed care has even greater market penetration than in the New York Metropolitan Region.

Data could be collected through interviews with the principals of IPAs and centers of excellence that employ multidisciplinary teams, as well as interviews with consumers; and by examining administrative information from IPAs and centers of excellence. The following topics need to be covered: (1) how negotiations were initiated and conducted, and with what results; (2) any changes in the kinds of services delivered to special needs populations; and (3) the extent to which service delivery has been improved by organizational redesigns and/or technologic enhancements introduced by managed care. In so doing, this type of study will permit planners and policy makers to determine if high-quality care for special needs populations is maintained or sacrificed in an age where cost drives service delivery.

PROGRAMS THAT SERVE PEOPLE WITH DISABILITIES

During the past two decades, disability advocates often saw professional service providers as adversaries because they limited the capacity of people with disabilities to obtain self-determination. Today, with managed care dominating the private insurance market, and the prospect of commercialized Medicaid managed care for the poor and individuals with disabilities waiting in the wings, a family-professional alliance to protect access to needed resources may be a more appealing definition of empowerment. Current efforts to create that kind of unity is beginning to emerge at academic medical centers. Once perceived as the enemy of empowerment by families of children with disabilities, the centers are now spearheading the fight to save Medicaid as we know it.

Public funding through the federal-state formula for Medicaid led to payment for many services vital to an improved quality of life for people with disabilities. Many of the kinds of services so important to children and adults with developmental disabilities are defined as "collateral" or "ancillary" therapies, reimbursed by Medicaid and health insurance. As a result, these labels and payment mechanisms are remote from the concerns of state officials who focus primarily on preserving the infrastructure of public health and acute care in their localities. Advocates of public budget restraint may argue against the use of the Medicaid and Medicare systems to pay for so many therapeutic, residential, or support services, but no other options are currently available or likely to be offered in the future. The adoption of the ICIDH-2 classification system by health service providers, researchers, and policy makers would create a strong justification for financing interventions that could reduce reliance on traditional medical care.

VIEWS FROM SOME STAKEHOLDERS

The professionals who provide highly specialized health services to the disabled are most sensitive to the changing financial picture brought about by the advent of managed care. Access to rehabilitation services is a major concern for people with disabilities. The providers of such care are well aware of the need to support inpatient rehabilitation, often costing $1,000 a day or more. Cost-containing MCOs have a great deal at stake in keeping people out of this form of care.

To determine the impact of managed care on these highly specialized centers, Gerben DeJong of the National Rehabilitation Hospital Research Center conducted a telephone survey of rehabilitation providers in three health care markets that are characterized by high market penetration by MCOs. For providers attempting to limit damage and restore functioning for a patient, the in-hospital acute care units would be the location of choice. However, in many instances managed care payers bypass inpatient rehabilitation altogether. They approve rehabilitation services, but in subacute care units only.

Given this trend, rehabilitation providers have linked up with larger health care systems to encourage referrals from acute-care hospitals. Cost cutting has called into question a valid and cherished way of developing a treatment plan—the interdisciplinary team approach whereby each discipline or department through weekly team meetings arrives at a plan of care. The give-and-take of these discussions may not be of value when the hospital is no longer the foundation of the rehabilitation service delivery system:

> With managed care, the fee for service and cost based methods of rehabilitation payment are vanishing rapidly, but full case-rate capitation has yet to come to rehabilitation in any significant way. Most acute and subacute rehabilitation providers in the three markets studied are being paid on a fixed per-diem basis, where length of stay is negotiated depending on patient status and progress. (DeJong, 1996: 138)

VIEWS FROM SOME STAKEHOLDERS CONTINUED

To what extent are these trends being felt in those centers of excellence that make up the network of University Affiliated Programs for People with Developmental Disabilities (UAPs) funded by the Federal Health and Human Services' Administration on Developmental Disabilities? Each UAP seeks to provide exemplary services, training, research and its dissemination, and technical assistance to other agencies in the community. In essence, a UAP is the bridge between the academic world and the community.

The evolution of this network mirrors some of the changes in the delivery of community care in the field of developmental disabilities. In 1963, with the passage of the Mental Retardation and Mental Health Community Facility Development Act (P.L. 88–164), the Kennedy administration and Congress created university-affiliated facilities that would be constructed to promote improved services and training in the field of mental retardation. Subsequent reauthorizations of this legislation, now more familiarly known as the Developmental Disabilities Act, broadened the scope of the initial law to include a range of developmental disabilities, currently defined in functional terms, and arranged to provide funding for UAPs. The latter legislation did not require the presence of a constructed facility, as mandated in the 1963 law, but only that a program fulfill the mandate requiring UAPs to provide training, technical assistance, dissemination of new findings, and, until recently, exemplary service activities. Services are now an optional activity, but one with which most UAPs are still involved. The first university-affiliated facilities were based in medical centers and most of these programs still are based there. In fact, 35 current UAPs receive funding from the federal Maternal and Child Health Bureau (MCHB) to provide leadership training in the care of children with neurodevelopmental disabilities and related disorders. This funding source requires an interdisciplinary (ID) training model to be based in both medical centers and in community settings.

As a result, the majority of UAPs provide significant health services as well as other services. UAPs often function as tertiary referral centers for diagnosis and treatment of children and, in some instances, adults with disabilities. In some programs, primary care is also delivered to clients.

What has evolved over the past three decades has been a network of UAPs with varied commitments to service activities, plus concomitant training, program development, technical assistance, and research and dissemination activities, often varying with the skills and interests of the faculty and the requirements of federal, state, or local funding sources. The latter may include contracts, demonstration projects, or grants. In sum, UAP service roles are often idiosyncratic to the particular university or locality. While each UAP is unique, those that depend on patient fees are most vulnerable to the growth of managed care.

To examine the impact of managed care directly on the delivery of services and the financial stability of UAPs, my colleague Herbert J. Cohen and I surveyed 61 members of the network in 1996. While there are 68 UAPs in the United States and its territories, we eliminated those that were clearly identified as not having substantial clinical components. From the remaining 61, another 12 wrote back to us that they did not provide clinical services and another 12 did not respond to two requests to complete the survey. With 49 UAPs then eligible for the survey, our response rate was 76 percent. A further review of the nonresponding UAPs revealed that less than half of the 12 that did not respond had a substantial clinical component.

The survey could be returned anonymously or the institution, and the person completing the survey, could be included, if so desired. Only two respondents decided to remain anonymous. Eleven of the 15 questions allowed for extended responses to support declarations concerning such recent or current topics such as:

- shifts in funding
- relationships with HMOs
- state efforts to declare UAPs as "essential community providers"

- special arrangements undertaken by state Medicaid to support services for people with development disabilities (DD)
- unintended consequences of the state shifting to Medicaid managed care
- the impact on training programs at the UAP and clinical activities
- the development of new alliances and partnerships
- staff reductions due to changes in service funding
- new efforts at marketing
- any hiring of management consulting firms
- predictions for future funding

What follows is a report on both the frequency distribution of answers by UAP directors to specific questions related to the above-cited topics and a few of their brief verbal descriptions and explanations of the impact of changing funding patterns for diagnostic evaluation and treatment. Finally, I suggest some recommendations for action for UAPs and their national association.

Results

Note that this effort was sparked by some of the disquieting trends shared among UAP directors at national meetings. Indeed, these anecdotal remarks were confirmed in the survey: 59 percent of the respondents said that there has been a significant shift during the past two years in funding of clinical services. One respondent described this change as creating "a wave of change within the insurance industry. The overall success of applying HMO concepts saves dollars, controls costs and eliminates the insurance 'middle man.' "

For one UAP in the Middle West the HMO movement was nothing new, since they have been living with them for over a decade. For that program, "the reduction of referrals due to HMOs has been significant over the past ten years. HMOs were first introduced as a major form of insurance in Wisconsin in the early 1980s."

Several other respondents attested to the reduction of referrals from primary care providers who cannot seek consultations out-of-plan. For those who do receive referrals, they note the substantial fee discounts demanded by HMOs to get referrals. One comment aptly summarized the new funding pattern:

As more people have enrolled in HMOs, we have noted more restrictions on services and poorer reimbursement rates. In some cases, disciplines have had difficulty receiving any reimbursement. Also many HMOs do not want to pay for interdisciplinary evaluations. HMOs want medical services only.

The concern was also expressed that quality was being affected by the conversion of Medicaid to managed care as well as in the commercial HMO. To save money, children were being sent to places where appropriate diagnostic testing and evaluations were not done and where they were receiving treatment based on inappropriate diagnoses. Part of the problem was due to less coverage of services by Medicaid under managed care.

The consequences for clinical programs not only mean fewer referrals to pediatric subspecialists but a shift from inpatient to outpatient care with less income. With a lower revenue base, there was an overall decline noted in providing uncompensated care. Moreover, changes in service funding was deemed responsible for a reduction in staff at 46 percent of the UAPs reporting.

UAPs were active in seeking to become players in this new game of managed care. Approximately half of the respondents have established contractual relations with HMOs or other managed care organizations, with either for-profit (4) or nonprofit organizations (6) or with both types (8). Five provided discounted fee-for-service, three had arrangements that mixed risk-based capitation and case rates, while only three were capitated.

It is evident from the survey that many UAPs were seeking stable sources of income. More interesting were the descriptions of these arrangements, sometimes part of AMC-driven contracts for provider groups with HMOs. Those UAPs that are not part of such contracts, while still part of AMCs, feel left out of plans and seek other partnerships.

There is little consistency found among the various partnerships and the payment systems described. What is paid for in one arrangement may not be paid for in another. Capitated rates may exist for the physician and psychologist but not for other allied health providers. Alternatively, in some cases there may be a fee-for-service packaged rate for a full interdisciplinary evaluation.

At this point in time, only five (14 percent) UAPs reported that discussions were underway with state agencies so that state regulations of HMOs would require that their programs be declared an "essential community provider" and that all HMOs serving special needs populations establish working agreements or contracts with them. Only one respondent reported that the state required these affiliations, but did not feel that the program worked: "All provider groups must provide a comprehensive package. Our Medicaid programs have strict working rules and more lax enforcement."

Conversion of state Medicaid to capitated risk-based managed care was reported by 17 UAP directors with an additional 10 stating that it will occur within one year. Only 10 (27 percent) said that it had not and would not occur presently in their states. Arrangements for special needs populations such as the developmentally disabled involved what is universally referred to as a "carve out." This means that fee-for-service payment and direct access to specialists will continue with, in some states, "HMOs being required to have arrangements with special needs providers." A few UAP directors reported that their diagnostic evaluation and therapeutic services would be subject to a rate-adjusted capitation payment for all medical services, including primary care.

Despite the frequently mentioned "carve outs," the conversion of state Medicaid to managed care has also produced unintended consequences for people with developmental disabilities, including the failure of primary care providers to acquire the appropriate medical training, knowledge of the system of services in place, and communication skills to work with patients with developmental disabilities. The low level of knowledge about the delivery system by case managers also was identified as a problem. However, one respondent believed that people with developmental disabilities were doing better than expected.

Only one-quarter of the sample said that training programs were affected by changes in funding due to the growth of managed care. As suspected, revenues from clinical programs had helped offset the costs of training programs in several locations. This now presents a problem in supporting teaching faculty who were required to be listed as trainers on grant applications, even though their funding came from other, that is, clinical, sources. A few respondents mentioned that they were seeking more training grants as a result of this decrease in funding. Several directors mentioned that managed care was now part of the training curriculum. One respondent also pointed out how community training was impacted by reductions in funding for clinical services:

> [There is a] definite increase in content material for trainees regarding managed care, HMOs, and new financing arrangements. We are seeing more in the out-patient department (OPD), therefore, [there is] less time available for our OPD staff (traditionally the ones to do community-based training) to get into communities to train. This is being recognized more and more by community-based agencies saying "where is the UAP help we previously had?"

This recognition of the unintended consequences of the growth of managed care also extended to perceived marginalization of the interdisciplinary approach taken at most UAPs: "Some HMOs will not cover the cost of an interdisciplinary assessment because they have all the individual professionals in their organization, although they do not work as a team."

One director suggested that the movement to managed care has forced UAPs to become more efficient in their use of resources. These comments make this UAP remarkably like the mirror image of an HMO.

> We have attempted to create clinical protocols that eliminate services of marginal diagnostic value. We are constantly reviewing lab tests ordered to use less expensive screens and eliminate testing that would be passed on to our patients.

In the face of reduced revenues, about half of the UAPs reported that they were developing new alliances and partnerships. Some of these arrangements were based on expansion of work with Early Intervention Services, school systems, state programs for children with special health care needs (Title V), and state mental retardation/developmental disability (MR/DD) agencies. Other alliances are with providers under contract with HMOs rather than direct contracts with HMOs. In some cases respondents noted that they were involved in many linkages at the same time. A few directors mentioned that they were starting innovative programs that would take them into the area of public health, for example, prevention and treatment of lead poisoning.

Through the development of brochures, new types of services, mailings, speakers bureaus, formal presentations to state officials, outreach educational programs, stories in the mass media, and physician education, over half the UAPs attempted to market themselves better than in the past. Increased visibility in the community was one objective of this effort with the ultimate goal being increased freedom from dependency on health care financing either through fees or capitation. One UAP director stated that his program was working with an internally devised plan:

> We named a definitive, experienced internal marketing group. They have devised a sophisticated marketing plan. We are providing educational material to all referring MDs with mailing of reports. As above, new Area Educational Agency relationship. We have initiated clinical evaluations with MDs in remote sites over the Iowa Communications Network (ICN), a hard wired fiber optic system covering the entire state. Physicians and community agencies love it. The "clinical thing of the future."

We asked whether outside help was sought. Only six UAPs used management consultants to assist in preparing for the new forms of financing, with no single objective in common. Revenue enhancement was mentioned as one goal, along with identifying how the UAP was perceived in the community. The efforts to gain greater control over the external environment by using consultants did not lead to immediate gains for the UAPs involved.

When asked to predict the funding picture for MR/DD clinical services in the next five years, 33 out of 37 ventured a guess. Adjectives such as "grim," "very difficult," "bleak," and "confused" were found often in describing the new restrictions on funding that came with the advent of managed care. Decreased referrals were often predicted. More federal intervention was suggested to create a safety net for the developmentally disabled. Cost containment was seen as driving the system and reducing quality, especially for a Medicaid-dependent population.

> The state's Medicaid population is in the process of being shifted to MCOs without special provisions for special needs population. We anticipate a significant reduction in referrals and reimbursement as well as limitations of services as a result of this shift. Medicaid tends to be the payer of last resort for individuals with MR/DD and their families and funds nearly 70% of the patient care at KKI. We are very concerned about a decline in service and quality of care for the special needs population.

What can we do to preserve rehabilitation hospitals' and UAPs' dedication to exemplary service, training, research, and technical assistance? It is these activities that give value to a national hospital or even a national network of programs.

First, serious educational work is required on the state level to remind legislators that cost containment has its consequences—not only in jobs lost but in the loss of critically needed specialized services for the developmentally disabled and their families that took decades to develop, as well as the destruction of programs that help create and develop new knowledge and that train the subspecialists whom we turn to in time of need. Furthermore, disabilities are found among all social classes. With the attempt to contain the rapid rise in health care costs of the past 10 years, which was slowing down without managed care, planners and policy makers may be destroying much-needed services. There is a communal imperative to sustain the programs that offer quality care for those with complex medical problems.

Second, cost should not drive quality out of health care. (Or to restructure a recent aphorism: The good should not be an enemy of the perfect.) We need to convince decision makers that the interdisciplinary approach is essential for providing care for adults with spinal cord injuries or identifying the scope and types of problems early in the life of a child with developmental disabilities. In the former case, intervention usually results in greater independence, integration, and productivity. In the latter case, early identification, intervention, and the prevention of secondary disabilities are cost effective. Placing a child in programs—and reducing the adverse impact of medical conditions—pays off by producing a more productive member of society while reducing opportunity costs for other members of the family.

Third, HMOs need to offer comprehensive services. Health care does not end with prevention and early intervention. The professionals who know something about disabilities should be required to be available to HMOs both to provide service and to train primary care providers about these conditions and their consequences. On a systems level, subspecialists should be involved actively in developing clinical practice guidelines for specific developmental disabilities to avoid useless or unnecessary therapies and promote the adoption of effective therapies. These subspecialists can be available on a contractual basis from rehabilitation hospitals or UAPs and trained in HMOs by hospital staff or UAP faculty.

UAPs and rehabilitation hospitals should be there to make sure that our world class medical care be available for all Americans—embedded in all delivery systems—and not be a memory to most and/or accessible only to rich, often foreign, patients who can afford it.

REFERENCES

Biles, B., and Simon, L. 1996. "Academic health centers in an era of managed care." *Bulletin of the New York Academy of Medicine* (Winter Supplement): 484–489.

Birenbaum, A., and Cohen, H. J. 1997. "Managed care and UAPs: Views from some stakeholders." Presented at the annual meeting of the American Association on Mental Retardation (May 30th), New York, NY.

DeJong, G. 1996. "Medical rehabilitation undergoing major shake up in advanced managed care markets." *Bureau of National Affairs' Managed Care Reporter* (February): 138–141.

Donelan, K., Blendon, R. J., Hill, C. A., Hoffman, C., Rowland, D., Frankel, M., and Altman, D. 1996. "Whatever happened to the health insurance crisis in the United States? Voices from a national survey." *Journal of the American Medical Association* 276 (October 23/30): 1346–1350.

Jensen, G. A., Morissey, M. A., Gaffney, S., and Liston, D. K. 1997. "The new dominance of managed care: Insurance trends in the 1990s." *Health Affairs* (January/February): 125–136.

8

Public Health Partnerships:
Work in Progress

For more than a century public health experts have recognized the impact on health and longevity of social and natural environmental factors (Epstein, 1998). These observations have become part of the conceptual apparatus of public health teaching and interventions. Called today "population-based health care," it is a translation of the public health view to the locus of health care delivery. This is no better expressed than in medical sociologist David Mechanic's understanding of health interventions:

> Health promotion and disease prevention depend on a population perspective that allows for the identification of risks and the mobilization of protective and remedial interventions for both the individual and the community. (1998: 874)

Some epidemiologists have argued recently that it is the *relative* differences within a society that encourage the development of chronic disease and higher accident rates as well as higher death rates among the poor (Wilkinson, 1996; Wolf and Bruhn, 1997). Thus the higher up one is on the social ladder, the less one is subject to stress and the lower the death rates on one's social stratum. Within the same regional population, there can be wide variations in rates of morbidity and mortality. Even more interesting and distressing is the fact that life expectancy differences between the rich and the poor are widening today. Death rates have declined rapidly among the higher social classes in the last three decades while they have shown no decline among the poorest sectors of society. Among the poor, the likelihood of an early death is dramatically higher than among the rich (Epstein, 1998: 27). Reducing infant mortality and the acquisition of life-long disabilities remains a targeted goal of public health agencies, particularly those targeted to improving a pregnant woman's prenatal and a newborn's postnatal care. Finally, for a variety of reasons having to do with the ecologic and social stresses undergone by poor people in our society, the rate of disability is higher among poor people than among those better off.

These health promotion and disease prevention perspectives were adopted by the Association of Maternal and Child Health Programs (AMCHP), an assembly of state Title V programs, in their 1996 mandate to establish cooperative relationships with managed care organizations as a first step in supporting and improving child health in the community. In so doing, AMCHP regarded managed care organizations as contributors to population-based efforts to improve health.

Managed care provides an opportunity to work toward mutually desired goals with public health organizations such as state maternal and child health programs. Mechanic notes that

> as medical care providers increasingly are paid by capitation and are more often evaluated according to their success in improving outcomes, public health efforts at the individual as well as the community level are in their interest. (1998: 874)

However, as Mechanic observes with some regret, the competition among plans in the marketplace does not create incentives to invest in community-wide programs that may benefit the plans' enrollees but is not exclusively limited to those enrollees. Increasingly, letting the marketplace provide health services for the majority of the population puts in jeopardy some of the safety net that was built during the Progressive Era, the New Deal, and the Great Society. It also limits support through cross-funding of some of the foundations of health care in the United States: medical education, research, and care for the uninsured (Birenbaum, 1997). In a profound sense, using the marketplace for health care reform may weaken the existing public health infrastructure that has taken almost a century to create.

At this time in the social history of the United States, there is more reason than ever before for the providers and public health agencies to see the benefits of mutual participation in improving the nation's health. The report of a major conference on this subject speaks to the power of collaboration and the material interest of providers in supporting the public health sector:

> As the medical sector takes on financial risk, it also becomes economically dependent on the public health sector, particularly on the capacity of public health agencies to prevent unnecessary disease from occurring in the community. Under capitation—in striking contrast to fee-for-service or cost-based payment—treating medical problems consumes the medical sector's resources instead of increasing its revenues. Consequently, in today's environment, managed care organizations and capitated medical practices bear the costs of treating patients who come down with diseases that occur when efforts to protect the community's food, water, housing, and environment fail. (Lasker, 1997: 37)

The history of the relationship between public health and medicine began as a mutually supportive relationship in the early twentieth century when medicine was attempting to gain legitimation. It encompassed the period of professionalization and the transformation of medical practice that focused on infectious diseases and acute care for the individual, and since World War II, there has been intensified separation of functions (Lasker, 1997: 7–8).

There was an extraordinarily uneven development of resources in the 1950s, which accelerated in the 1960s.

> Reflecting public demand for biomedical advances, funding was considerably less generous for population-based public health programs than for medical care; for health departments than for hospitals; for epidemiologic and social science investigation than for clinical studies and basic science research; and for the education and training of public health professionals than for those in medicine. In 1990, 2.7 percent of the nation's health dollars went for public health. (Lasker, 1997: 19)

There is good reason to believe that the individualistic culture of American society helps sustain this disparity. What is done for us all gets eclipsed by the drama of medical care for the person dealing with accident or disease.

> Medical care does well in a free-market economy like the United States because it is closely tied to individuals; the benefits of seeing a medical practitioner are realized directly by the individual receiving care. In public health, on the other hand, the benefits of community-wide strategies to prevent disease and promote health are received by everyone, including people who do not pay for them directly. (Lasker, 1997: 19)

In addition to preventive efforts, the state and federal governments often have used tax revenues to provide for services that individuals or families cannot afford to pay for. State legislatures have established special funds for hemophiliacs so that expensive blood products could be purchased by families of modest means. Long before these dedicated programs of financing were developed, federal legislation created the mechanisms to assist families with children with major medical expenses.

ORIGINS OF TITLE V

The establishment of Social Security was a landmark in American social history, not just because of the pensions now available for retired workers and their beneficiaries, but because it addressed some of the major health needs of all children through programs in all the states and territories. Welfare services for children needing special care and maternal and child health services, including services for "crippled children," were enacted in 1935 as Title V of the Social Security Act. In essence, Title V established a formula under which states received grants to create units to develop and direct clinical preventive health services for the broad population of mothers and children and medical services for children with special health care needs, referred to as "crippled children" in the original legislation (Hutchins, 1997).

The first recognition that children deserved special attention by the national government actually was mandated a quarter-century earlier. The Children's Bureau was a federal agency established by Congress in 1912 and signed into law by President William Howard Taft. Under the guidance of the bureau and its successor agencies, state Title V programs have made significant advances in children's health over the past 60 years, including creating access for children with special health care needs to complex medical care and durable medical equipment. Title V agencies also perform public health functions by designing and implementing "systems of care to improve the health and well-being of children and their families in local communities" (Hayes and Walker, 1997: 344).

The state Title V programs were concerned during the 1990s that some of the public health functions performed by providers might be eliminated with the growth of health plans that strictly defined benefits for enrollees. The Association of Maternal and Child Health Programs (1996) recommended recently that "managed care arrangements should work collaboratively with the health system infrastructure on a local and state level to determine how it can best be integrated into that system to support and complement community level population-based efforts to improve health." To what extent has this integration taken place?

In the winter of 1998, I surveyed 57 programs in all the states and territories. This inquiry received 39 replies, or a response rate of 68 percent, to my request for information about discussions, proposals and collaborations with either for-profit or nonprofit managed care organizations (MCOs). From that total of 39 replies, I found that 23 programs, or 58 percent, had some kind of contact with MCOs. Most of the others, 42 percent, were in states where the managed care market penetration was extremely low.

The numeric responses ranged from the quantifiable to the unquantifiable (e.g., "too many to count"), particularly in regard to the question concerning discussions and to a lesser extent with regard to proposals. Respondents also made several comments about the futility of attempting to measure quantifiably relationships between MCOs and Title V programs. These same respondents, to their credit, were willing to provide detailed descriptions of the collaborations established between their agency and MCOs.

Nine Title V programs, generally from the prairie states, wrote that there was no managed care in their states and they, therefore, could not complete the survey. Among those answering that there was some managed care presence in their state (n=30), we found a number of collaborations in place in 1996 and in 1997. Twenty-three programs reported at least one discussion in their state or one proposal made, sometimes even without discussion taking place.

For the states that had collaborative projects with nonprofit MCOs, there was an almost one-to-one correlation (0.95) between those Maternal and Child Health (MCH) programs that had projects in 1996 and those that had them in 1997. There was only a partial correlation (0.35) for the states that reported on collaborations with for-profit MCOs, meaning that there was a great deal of turnover from category to category when the two years are compared. Moreover, there was a slight negative correlation for 1996 and a slight positive correlation for 1997 between collaborations with both for-profit and nonprofit organizations in the same year (−0.13; 0.16), demonstrating that state MCH programs had modest overlap in involvement in both types of MCOs.

As can be seen in Table 3, for both years there were more collaborations listed with nonprofit than for-profit managed care organizations. The mean number of collaborations with for-profit MCOs was significantly fewer when compared to collaborations with non-profit MCOs. Second, the percentage of nonprofit collaborations increased modestly from 39 percent in 1996 to 45.6 percent. Moreover, the mean number of collabora-

Table 3
**Number and Percentage of Collaborations with For-profit and
Nonprofit Managed Care Organizations (N=23)**

	For-profit		Nonprofit	
1996	0	78.3%	0	60.9%
	1–3	21.7%	1–4	39.1%
	mean=.478		mean=1.26	
1997	0	82.6%	0	54.5%
	2	13.0%	1	9.1%
	7	4.3%	2–4	27.5%
			10	4.5%
			30	4.5%
	mean=.565		mean=2.63	

tions with nonprofit MCOs per reporting program increased substantially
from 1.26 in 1996 to 2.63 in 1997.

TECHNICAL ASSISTANCE FOR THE STATE
MEDICAID AGENCY

The major role reportedly played by the Title V programs related to assisting the states' departments of health, or in some cases departments of
public welfare, in preparing and organizing the requests for proposals or applications for Medicaid managed care contracts. They performed this technical assistance role in a number of ways.

- The Title V agencies established the criteria for adequate capacity for maternal
  and child health services that would have to be written into managed care contracts.
- They reviewed applications received by the Medicaid agency in six states.
- They reviewed the memoranda of understanding that were established between
  local health departments and MCOs regarding maternal and child health services.

The state maternal and child health agencies or, in the most populated
states such as California, local health agencies also provided services that
were purchased directly by the MCOs. Public health services targeted to
women and children were offered by the public health agencies and paid

for by the MCOs. In Hawaii, the maternal and child health agency provided services to high-risk pregnant women that were reimbursed through contacts with MCOs. Subsequently, this state's Title V agency prepared a prenatal case management model that was purchased by MCOs.

Standards for prenatal care programs, including protocols, were produced by the state agency for use by Medicaid managed care programs in West Virginia. Discussions between the Title V program and MCOs about services that could be delivered by the state agency were identified in the surveys. In Massachusetts, the agency works with the MCOs in relation to early intervention infant services. The MCOs have formal representation on the state interagency coordinating council.

In Oregon the state maternal and child health agency also brokered the creation of contracts between school-based health centers (SBHC) and Medicaid managed care providers so the MCOs could be charged for the services rendered. Similarly, in Connecticut, the Title V agency collaborated with the state Medicaid agency to get SBHCs recognized as Medicaid providers and consequently eligible to be participating providers in Medicaid managed care.

Partnering also took place, without service purchases, in the organization of an immunization registry, school health programs, and pre- and postnatal home visiting, with the Title V program monitoring the referral process when early intervention services were warranted.

QUALITY ASSURANCE AND IMPROVEMENT

In the language of total quality management (TQM), programs need models to emulate. A consistent standard to be matched or striven for is called a benchmark. Title V agencies sought to raise the standard of performance of MCOs serving the Medicaid-eligible part of the population by setting goals to be met in immunization. They sought to hold MCOs to high standards of performance even when it was feared that these standards might scare away vendors.

Queries about population-based initiatives elicited responses that went beyond direct work with MCOs. The Title V agencies also mentioned organized public health campaigns in their states to reduce teenage pregnancy, domestic violence, and smoking, while increasing access to prenatal care.

There was particular concern among our respondents that the children with special health care needs (CSHCN) might not receive high quality services in Medicaid managed care plans. The Family Health Issues Partnership Plan Implementation Subcommittee, New York State Department of Health, defines CSHCN according to the presence of chronic conditions that require additional services. They are

> those children (0–21 years) who have or are suspected of having a serious or chronic physical, developmental, behavioral, or emotional condition and who also require health and related services of type or amount beyond that required by children generally. (New York State Department of Health, 1997)

Discussions took place in several states about how to improve these services through better care coordination. One respondent replied that the agency was "currently drafting a memorandum of understanding between our CSHCN program, our EPSDT outreach and case management program and one MCO, which is to serve as a model for replication."

Quality improvement also extends to staff development. The Ohio Title V agency, along with the Ohio Association of Health Plans, held seven information-sharing sessions for public health nurses, primary care providers, service coordinators, parents, and local HMO representatives.

State Medicaid agencies can also be leaders in partnerships, encouraging seamless care for children with special needs. In Cleveland, a partnership called Access Better Care (ABC) formed a comprehensive, interdisciplinary program for children with developmental disabilities. This began as a joint effort between a for-profit managed care company, a medical center under contact with the Ohio Department of Human Services, and the state Medicaid agency (Brooks, 1997: 362).

Capitation was paid for by the Ohio Department of Human Services to United HealthCare, the for-profit managed care company, through a tiered capitation program, based on the utilization of services for the child in the previous year. A complex financial formula protects the MCO against excessive losses in providing care for a child.

The medical care was under the control of a pediatrician and there were no prior authorization requirements for referrals for subspeciality providers. All subspecialty providers were compensated on a fee-for-service basis. Their fees were beyond the usual Medicaid fee and they also received additional fees for care coordination.

There is a sad ending to this promising project, evident by the use of the past tense to refer to activities at ABC. Despite what appeared to be excellent services provided and outcomes for the children receiving care through ABC, United HealthCare found that it was losing money on the project and withdrew in November 1997, effectively ending the experiment in cooperation between a state Medicaid agency, a full-service provider, and a for-profit MCO.

FUTURE ROLES

In addition to attempts to develop standards and to implement quality assurance measures in state contracts with MCOs, it is clear that the Title V program will have to assume an active role in order to guarantee satisfactory services for CSHCNs. These functions include: advocacy and/or a requirement for making direct arrangements for training for primary care providers in managed care systems to become more familiar with the needs of CSHCNs and their families; facilitating the development of practice guidelines for services for specific common disorders or disabilities in the CSHCN population; and implementing a data collection system to track the outcomes and followup on the disposition of CSHCNs in the managed care system.

The network of state maternal and child health programs, along with the federal funding agency, the Maternal and Child Health-Bureau, have become interested in the ways in which MCOs could utilize the HEDIS 3.0 evaluation tool, as described in chapter 6, to demonstrate whether services to CSHCNs are adequate under these new forms of health care financing and delivery. By funding projects to monitor managed care, the Maternal and Child Health-Bureau is essentially gathering information nationally and uses experts on health care for children with chronic conditions to make recommendations to ensure quality care. This team has argued for implementation of specific steps to assure quality within and across managed care plans (Kuhlthau et al., 1998).

First, there is a need to create a mechanism to identify this population. Data collected for administrative purposes could be used, making for modest expenditures. Data collection efforts from families upon enrollment as part of the intake process or following major medical events would be more costly. Claims or clinical records could be examined. This team of experts (Kuhlthau et al., 1998) note that

> other promising approaches include measures that combine functioning, severity and service need. These approaches determine whether the child has a chronic condition and then its effects in such areas as the child's usual activities or need for additional services. (49)

It is important that a single method of defining children with chronic conditions, using functional criteria, be used by all interested parties, and that it become part of the next version of HEDIS. Again, the ICIDH-2 offers a classificatory scheme that measures disability independent of health condition, undifferentiated by etiology, and features a full range of activities performed by a child within a gamut of social contexts. Its use would make it possible to determine with accuracy the level of severity of impairment and what steps need to be taken to maximize the child's full potential.

Second, HEDIS should be applied to all children, permitting a comparison on service utilization both for those with chronic conditions and those without. Preventive care, often a routine activity for children without chronic conditions, may become less certain for CSHCNs. Responsibility for the scheduling and performance of this activity may not be clear to all the specialty care providers who are dealing with complex medical procedures.

Third, building on the Consumer Assessment of Health Plans Survey (CAHPS) approach, the team recommends period surveys of parents of children with chronic conditions to provide information to the plans. In so doing, plans will learn whether parents think the services available are adequate to meet their needs. The question of how well the health services provided by the MCO are able to coordinate with other agencies such as school is important to address in a parent survey. They also recommend an independently conducted survey of the primary care physicians who have coordinative responsibility for CSHCNs to determine whether, in their view, access to pediatric subspecialists, mental health providers, and rehabilitation therapies is adequate.

Finally, Karen Kuhlthau and her colleagues also call for the development of structure, process, and outcome indicators specific to children with special health care needs. While these measures are the standards used in quality assurance in health care, there is a willingness among these experts to admit that the gold standard of outcome measures related to improvements in child functioning is limited at this time, although some promising scales exist.

Structural measures should focus on staffing—the access to specialized therapists, durable medical equipment, and mental health therapists. Additionally, there should be mechanisms in place to make the plan easy to use for parents of CSHCNs.

Process measures should include how well the provision of care matches quality-of-care protocols. "In addition, it should measure the extent to which services are comprehensive, coordinated, continuous, prevention oriented, family centered, and culturally competent" (Kuhlthau et al., 1998: 51). Outcome measures for a cross-section of children with chronic conditions are a dream. For specific conditions, the statistical problems associated with low prevalence makes outcome indicators suspect.

REFERENCES

Association of Maternal and Child Health Programs. 1996. "Partnerships for healthier families: Principles for assuring the health of women, infants, children, and young under managed care arrangements." Unpublished paper. Washington, DC: AMCHP.

Birenbaum, A. 1997. "Academic medical centers and the cost of managed care." *The Einstein Quarterly Journal of Biology and Medicine* 14 (3): 98–99.

Brooks, P. 1997. "Models of collaboration: Strategies for improving children's health in a managed care environment." In R.E.K. Stein, editor, *Health Care for Children: What's Right, What's Wrong, What's Next.* New York: United Hospital Fund of New York.

Epstein, H. 1998. "Life and death on the social ladder." *New York Review* 45 (July 16th): 26–30.

Hayes, M., and Walker, D. K. 1997. "The role of public health in assuring a system of health care for children." In R.E.K. Stein, editor, *Health Care for Children: What's Right, What's Wrong, What's Next.* New York: United Hospital Fund of New York.

Hutchins, V. L. 1997. "A history of child health and pediatrics in the United States." In R.E.K. Stein, editor, *Health Care for Children: What's Right, What's Wrong, What's Next.* New York: United Hospital Fund of New York.

Kuhlthau, K., Walker, D. K., Perrin, J. M., Bauman, L., Gortmaker, S. L., Newacheck, P. W., and Stein, E. K. 1998. "Assessing managed care for children with chronic conditions: New recommendations for monitoring care as increasing numbers of children with chronic conditions join managed care plans." *Health Affairs* 17 (July/August): 42–52.

Lasker, R. D. 1997. *Medicine and Public Health: The Power of Collaboration.* New York: The New York Academy of Medicine.

Mechanic, D. 1998. "Topics for our times: Managed care and public health opportunities." *American Journal of Public Health* 88 (June): 874–875.

New York State Department of Health. 1997. "Children with Special Health Care Needs Work Group executive summary and report." Unpublished paper. Albany: New York State Department of Health.

Wilkinson, R. G. 1996. *Unhealthy Societies: The Affliction of Inequality.* New York: Routledge.

Wolf, S., and Bruhn, J. G. 1997. *The Power of the Clan: The Influence of Human Relationships on Heart Disease.* New Brunswick, NJ: Transaction Press.

9

Protecting the Rights of Consumers

The introduction of managed care has contributed greatly to the reduced power and status of the medical profession in American society. Today doctors complain in public opinion polls that their work is less satisfying, their incomes reduced, and their efforts more entangled in paperwork to justify what they do. They do not recommend that their daughters and sons follow in their footsteps. Astonishingly, they report more back pain than in the past, while hardly engaging more frequently in heavy lifting! Are consumers sharing this pain? When subject to organizational rules in managed care organizations, providers acknowledge that they may be led to compromising the care that they give to patients.

The diminishing autonomy of providers is reflected in their inability to recommend and perform procedures without receiving prior authorization, the monitoring of primary care providers' referral patterns to specialists, and the slowed down acceptance of newly developed technologies and complex and expensive procedures. The fee-for-service payment system encouraged voluminous utilization, even where some of the procedures were unnecessary and potentially harmful to patients.

Payments for specialty care and the extensive use of inpatient treatment were subject to insignificant self-restraint and ineffective regulation up to about 1985—the point in time when a congressionally enacted law mandating the prospective payment system for in-hospital stays for Medicare-eligible patients started to take effect. Not all of the overpayment for the use of hospital time was socially unproductive. The surpluses above costs accrued by academic medical centers helped to support medical research and training of new doctors. Insofar as these tasks are not done, there may be a lessening of the health care system's capacity to provide more effective care.

The pain felt by the consumer may not be directly correlated with the shift from fee-for-service to capitation. Consumers do save money in relying on managed care because they have no deductibles and modest co-payments for office visits. For those people who are disproportionate users of health care services because they are suffering from serious chronic illnesses or disabilities, the savings would be very impressive when out-of-pocket costs are compared with indemnity insurance coverage.

Why then are consumers seeking protection in the form of legislation both on the state and federal levels? Why have state lawmakers been willing to pass consumer rights legislation, including protection of the right to sue an HMO? What kinds of protections are likely for Medicare- and Medicaid-eligible individuals, among whom are a disproportionate number of people with disabilities? Why is federal legislation for protection of privately insured consumers being considered?

As I attempt to answer these questions, I will try to do so in terms of which forms of protection are most salient to people with disabilities. This means that some more general protections such as full disclosure of how doctors are compensated will be discussed from the perspective of how they might impact on disproportionately high users of health care.

Before we examine this problem from the point of view of federal legislation, let us look at the states. The states have grown in power as the federal government has been downsized during the Clinton years. When right-wing conservatives (and some moderates) say that some problems are best solved at the state level, they are pointing to the fact that members of state legislatures are very sensitive to pressures from consumers, as well as doctors and other small business elites. Not needing a great deal of funding to run for state assemblies and senates, these office holders get elected by pressing the flesh of thousands of voters and providing immediate responses to problems raised during these encounters along with phone calls and letters from constituents.

In turn, state laws designed to protect some interest group can make a state hostile territory to a particular type of business. Nothing can produce more consternation in the hearts and minds of large corporations with production capacity or sales rooms in many states than the efforts of state legislators to regulate their businesses. These regulatory statutes make executives develop unique rules and operating procedures, stress the need to acquire certain kinds of hires, and require other kinds of activities not found in other states. Legislative liaisons from the corporate world spend a great deal of their time in state capitals attempting to block change rather than encouraging it. State legislation can be geared to making things difficult for certain businesses, thereby discouraging them from entering the state or expanding their operations.

Therefore, much of the change introduced on the state level is in the form of protectionist legislation. There are also possibilities for creating new ways of doing things. Many of the New Deal programs of President Franklin D. Roosevelt were first introduced in New York State when Al Smith was governor. In dealing with crises, states also can introduce major efforts to implement certain health policies, for example, universal coverage, using the resources at their disposal. Efforts of this kind are watched closely by federal officials and the governors of other states to see if this "laboratory experiment" will really work.

Policy-oriented foundations also watch the states closely. An enumeration of consumer protections for all 50 states was performed by Families USA Foundation, a liberal advocacy organization based in Washington, D.C. The report identified the 13 areas of protection listed below as being important to consumers. They are presented here as the foundation wrote them, in clear and simple language. I have listed next to each protection the number of states that have passed legislation regarding that specific protection, as of July 1998.

- the right to go to an emergency room and have the managed care plan pay for the resulting care, if a person reasonably believes he or she is experiencing an emergency—*31*

- the right to receive health care from an out-of-network provider when the health plan's network of providers is inadequate—*15*

- the right of a person with a serious illness or disability to use a specialist as a primary care provider—*10*

- the right of a seriously ill person to receive standing referrals to health specialists—*12*

- a woman's right to gain direct access to an obstetrician or gynecologist—*31*

- the right of a seriously ill patient or pregnant woman to continue receiving health care for a specified period of time from a physician who has been dropped by the health plan—*14*

- the establishment of a procedure that enables a patient to obtain specific prescription drugs that are not on a health plan's drug formulary—*8*

- the right to appeal denials of care through a review process that is external and independent of health plans—*15*

- the establishment of consumer assistance, or ombudsman, programs—*2*

- prohibitions against plans' use of so called "gag rules"—rules that prevent physicians and health providers from fully disclosing treatment options to patients—*45*

- prohibitions on plans' reliance on inappropriate financial incentives to deny or reduce necessary health care—*19*

- the establishment of state laws that prevent plans from prohibiting participation in clinical trials—*3*

- the establishment of state laws enabling enrollees to sue their health plans when they improperly deny care—*2*

This is a comprehensive list of protections. Further analysis, however, reveals the wide variation that exists among the states as far as efforts to regulate managed care are concerned. Vermont leads the nation with protection in 11 areas. Every state, with the exception of South Dakota, has at least one law regarding at least one of the above-cited protections of consumers. Many of these protections were made into law during the years 1997 and 1998. To what extent have consumers taken advantage of these new protections?

Health policy reporter Peter Kilborn found in late 1998 that complaints about HMOs have grown. Using data from health insurance regulators from 12 populous states with heavy concentrations of managed care, he found that conflicts "over denials and delay of care and over medication and forms of treatment" (1998: 22) have increased 50 percent over the last one to three years. Most of these disputes have been settled in favor of consumers and doctors. Some of the reversals of medical decisions involve instances where a consumer has been discharged from a hospital earlier than warranted by professional opinion, or when a new subscriber was denied access to the doctor who treated him or her before enrollment because the doctor was not part of the plan. In these instances case managers or patient representatives are able to intervene without using formal grievance procedures.

The reasons for the increase in complaints seem to have less to do with deterioration in the managed care system than the fact that consumers are getting up to speed on how to use the complaint and grievance system that is in place. An increase in the number of formal disputes reported may also be attributed to the fact that 17 states have working nonpartisan arbitration boards to which complaints may be channeled.

In time, the rate of complaints may drop, as they have in Minnesota, a state with 20 years of experience with HMOs and extremely tight regulation of these plans. Easy access to a "help" number for the Department of Health, the agency that regulates MCOs in Minnesota, may help to explain why plans may be reluctant to restrict services in an arbitrary fashion.

Following his re-election on March 26, 1997, President Clinton appointed the Advisory Commission on Consumer Protection and Quality in the Health Care Industry. The commission included 34 members from a wide variety of backgrounds, including consumers, business, labor, health care providers and health plans, state and local governments, and health care quality experts. On December 8, 1997, they reported their findings, recommending the passage of a federal consumer bill of rights and responsibilities. Many of the advisory commission's recommendations correspond to the protections found in state legislation.

Some of these protections could become enacted through regulations associated with the administration of federal programs. On September 17, 1998, President Clinton announced that new rules would protect Medicaid patients, and would take effect in late 1998 or early 1999. The president described his action as the appropriate response to the problems and abuses cited by the commission. These efforts at regulation to provide consumers with protection also are similar to the 13 protections presented in the analysis of state legislative actions (Pear, 1998a). Since a disproportionate number of people with disabilities receive Medicaid benefits, these administrative regulations should be welcome. They include assurances that the HMO has an adequate number of medical specialists to meet members' needs, allowing individuals with chronic or severe conditions to go directly to specialists, an anti-"gag-rule" prohibition, and the right of appeal both within the HMO and through an independent body of denials, limits, or ending of coverage of services. In addition, consumers must receive simply written and easily understood information about how the plan works and a list of participating doctors and hospitals. Choice of plans is also required.

Responding to the outrage expressed by many consumers who have recounted and complained before Congress about the failure of MCOs to provide them with quality care, usually involving a denial of benefits, especially when faced with a serious illness, a range of legislation was introduced in the House of Representatives in 1997. Even some Republican members of Congress, such as Georgia Representative Charlie Norwood, usually seen as the friends of big business, introduced legislation that not only sought independent review for consumers, but also would permit them to sue health plans and businesses that were self-insured under the

Federal Employee Retirement Income Security Act (ERISA) for personal injury or wrongful death.

Employers fear that allowing lawsuits for these reasons will increase their costs for health plans as well as their legal costs involved in defending themselves against being named by plaintiffs in civil actions. This effort to remove protection from unlimited liability for damages distinguishes the proposed legislation sponsored by Senate Democrats (Senate Bill 1890) from a Republican alternative (Senate Bill 2330). The GOP bill establishes reviews and limited liability for ERISA plans that deny investigational treatments for life-threatening illnesses.

The Senate Democrats in October 1998 made an effort to have the full Senate debate their bill to define patients' rights and to regulate managed care organizations. By a narrow vote, 50–47, the Senate rejected this effort to place consumer and provider rights on their legislative agenda.

With the country in the midst of the impeachment of a president for lying about his sexual liaisons with a young woman intern at the White House, the Democratic sponsors attempted to move forward incrementally on health care reform. What they were unable to do was to mount a serious consumer-backed campaign for this kind of legislation, despite the rising number of complaints about service denials.

In contrast, the lobbying efforts of the managed care industry, led by the well-funded Health Benefits Coalition, helped to sweep away any possible protections for consumers that would have substantial financial penalties for recovering damages for improper denial of care (Pear, 1998b). The industry-led public relations effort started in late January when the president's legal problems appeared to be serious. Advocates for no action on patient rights took advantage of this unique situation, and, at least in 1998, there were no federal protections.

In late 1998 there were still some GOP efforts to create a bill of rights in health care, albeit with fewer financial sanctions for MCOs. A Republican House of Representatives bill (4250) set up penalties for an ERISA health plan that disregards an independent review and loses in court. This legislation sets caps ($250,000) on punitive damages and for pain and suffering awards stemming from malpractice suits. The bill, sponsored by the Republican House leadership, was passed by the House of Representatives and sent to the Senate in the summer of 1998.

This major legislation would have made only minor changes in the practices of HMOs. There are additional modest consumer protections found in the bill, including those requiring doctors to tell patients about treatment options, allowing women to use an obstetrician-gynecologist as their primary care doctor, requiring MCOs to disclose information about costs, benefits, and performance, creating point-of-service options for all plans offered by employers, and requiring that all plans cover some emergency care.

The legislation proposed has been analyzed by both the Congressional Budget Office (CBO) and accounting firms to determine whether premiums would increase, given these additional consumer protections. The CBO estimated that liability provisions would increase premiums a modest 1.2 percent while the report from the Barents Group of KPMG Peat Marwick, consultant to the American Association of Health Plans, predicted an increase of 8.6 percent. The Barents report also predicted that employers would drop coverage for 1.8 million Americans if these provisions became law (Cropper, 1998).

As in the past, some state legislatures have foreshadowed efforts on the federal level. Texas, with its liability law in place for a year, found that not a single suit has been filed and that actual cost increases were only one-tenth of one percent (Cropper, 1998), well below the projected costs of the CBO and the Barents group for the Senate Democrats' bill.

With this partial evidence in place from Texas, with its huge population, it appears that the right to sue is not a great burden on payers and it encourages MCOs to be careful in decisions that impact on enrollees' lives. In turn, enforcement in the courts remains a right for consumers who feel that they have been wronged by management practices that strongly shape the way health care is delivered. HMOs and other managed care plans are not comfortable about being held accountable for treatment decisions with regard to a particular patient. Yet they need to be monitored and held accountable for errors involving undertreatment as well as the less expected occasions in managed care of overtreatment.

I would imagine that there are very few occasions where the MCOs undertreat. While this is reassuring, the public perception is that the plan may not be there for the person with a serious life-threatening condition because the costs of care may be extremely high. Consumers may be on to something. It is not the cost of a single complex medical treatment that concerns the accountants at the MCO but multiple treatments, disproportionate to the expected frequency in the lives covered by the plan.

This kind of situation is so threatening to the financial well-being of an MCO that some chief operating officers have been willing to pay for an expensive procedure, for example, a liver transplant, so long as the patient and the family are willing to take vows of silence. A plan's stewards do not want it to be known that they are soft-hearted, fearing that they will attract others with previously existing conditions that will have to be paid for and will create a very unhealthy medical-loss ratio (Trafford, 1998).

Perhaps the most comprehensive protections offered for consumers are being considered by the Health Care Financing Administration (HCFA), that branch of the Social Security Administration that supervises and directs Medicare and Medicaid. As the payer for both fee-for-service and the managed care versions of these two public insurance programs, HCFA has continued to seek better value for the health care dollars spent by the agency. This concern over value—an admixture of price and quality—has led the HCFA to promulgate rules to structure how states are to engage in paying for and regulating Medicaid managed care. Its proposed rules, printed in the *Federal Register* on September 19, 1998, not only establish patient rights but also mandate the state Medicaid agency to set up standards for the selection and performance of MCOs. These protections will extend to the 15 million Americans now covered by Medicaid.

The regulations go out of their way to affirm the dignity of the enrollee through establishing the right to information regarding his or her health care and access to health care. An individual in Medicaid managed care is to be treated with respect and there should be consideration for the enrollee's dignity and privacy. Access to one's records is also a right, along with the right to receive information on available treatment options and alternative courses of care.

While no longer insisting that no more than 75 percent of the enrollees in an MCO be Medicaid or Medicare beneficiaries, once established as a way of protecting publicly insured enrollees from being ghettoized, there are many protections that come right out of the playbook of consumers in privately insured managed care. Others are more in line with making sure that quality and capacity exist in these managed care plans. These include, in a brief sketch, the following protections:

- the application of the "prudent layperson's" standard when it comes to using emergency services; standards to determine whether emergency room use by a beneficiary was appropriate;

- criteria for showing adequate capacity and services;

- procedures for dealing with disputes between enrollees and the plan, including a complaint process, a grievance process, and a link to a fair-hearing process;

- protection for enrollees against liability for payment of an organization's or provider's debts in the case of insolvency;

- prohibitions against certain physician incentive payments;

- the development and implementation by state agencies of quality assessment and improvement strategies for their managed care arrangements;

- provisions for external and independent review of managed care activities, but compensation for utilization management activities cannot be structured so as to provide incentives for the denial, limitation, or discontinuation of medically necessary services;

- restrictions on marketing and sanctions when a plan is not in compliance with state standards;

- requirements that enrollment notices and informational and instructional materials relating to enrollment be provided in a manner and form that are easily understood by Medicaid enrollees and potential enrollees;

- an MCO may not establish restrictions that interfere with enrollee-practitioner communications, including the opportunity to receive from their health care providers the full range of medical advice and counseling appropriate for their conditions; and

- a system of sanctions, including fines, for MCOs that fail to provide medically necessary items and services that are required, impose excess premiums, put in place any act to discriminate against enrollees on the basis of health status, are involved in a misrepresentation or falsification of information to HCFA, the state agency, or enrollees, and fail to comply with the physician incentive requirements.

What HCFA intends to do is to extend through regulation a uniform national standard on quality of care for all enrollees. It will do this based on the knowledge and best practices derived from the first-generation managed care plans for the Medicaid-eligible. Evidence-based clinical-practice guidelines are to be employed in all MCOs. Minimum performance levels are required, with MCOs using standard measures required by state Medicaid agencies. State agencies may require MCOs to undertake specific performance improvement projects. Given that millions of Americans are now covered by Medicaid managed care, we now have an excellent opportunity to study how managed care functions when quality and capacity concerns are subject to regulatory control.

While there is a statutory exclusion of special populations from managed care, there is also a willingness to allow states to engage in mandatory enrollment for these groups. Included in this category are those eligible for Social Security Income benefits, those in foster care or other out-of-home placement, or those receiving foster care or adoption assistance. If exemptions were removed for any of these special populations, a state agency would be required to demonstrate how the individuals' special needs and circumstances would be met under the managed care arrangements. There is a growing body of state experience and best practices regarding enrollment of these groups. We will use this knowledge when evaluating whether a particular state's waiver request does demonstrate that their program will adequately address the needs and complexities of these groups that set them apart from the groups that can be mandatorily enrolled without a waiver. (Health Care Financing Administration, 1998: 52032)

Of particular concern for people with disabilities, who are disproportionately found as enrollees in Medicaid, are the following items in the proposed regulation. It mentioned that access to specialty services is part of the general capacity of each MCO. Each MCO that seeks to serve Medicaid beneficiaries is required to submit documentation of its capacity to serve the expected enrollment in its service area. Moreover, there should be sufficient flexibility in the MCO's capacity to meet significant changes in the enrollee population. Finally, each state agency would be required to ensure that all covered services are available and accessible to enrollees. In particular,

> state agencies and MCOs should consider whether or not facilities are physically accessible when reviewing the MCO's delivery network. Enrollees with disabilities should have an appropriate choice of accessible providers. (Health Care Financing Administration, 1998: 52043)

The provision of services is to be monitored through such techniques as a member survey, analysis of member complaints and grievances, provider self-reports on waiting time, supplemented by random phone calls to consumers, test calls, and establishment of the rate at which enrollees abandon their efforts to reach an MCO representative by phone.

It has often been suggested that MCOs should pay close attention to people with disabilities. The new regulation also proposes that MCOs must provide an initial assessment of each enrollee's health within 90 days of enrollment and even shorter periods for individuals with complex and serious medical conditions.

The monitoring of individuals at-risk does not stop with the initial screening. The regulation also emphasizes that there should be current treatment plans for individuals with disabilities or other serious conditions. Medicaid beneficiaries with complex and serious medical conditions should also have direct access to specialists within the network for an appropriate number of visits under a plan of treatment. Two of the examples given follow:

> [a] multiple sclerosis patient under an approved treatment plan with a sacral decubitus who is referred to a specialist within the network for surgical debridement and wound care; or a situationally depressed patient under an

approved treatment plan who is referred to a specialist within the network for a course of therapy. (Health Care Financing Administration, 1998: 52044–52045)

Care coordination is not just recommended but required when dealing with complex and serious conditions. A single health professional or a team of providers, having primary responsibility for evaluating the enrollee's needs, is to orchestrate services. This includes recommendations and the arrangement of services required by the person.

While special populations may be eligible for services, they are not mentioned among the potential board members for the Medical Advisory Committee that each state must establish as a source of consultation with consumers and providers. While consumers' groups such as Medicaid recipients and consumer organizations such as labor unions are mentioned, disability advocates are not (see 52036).

REFERENCES

Cropper, C. M. 1998. "In Texas, a laboratory test on the effects of suing H.M.O.s." *New York Times* (September 13th): Business Section, pp. 1, 9.

Health Care Financing Administration. 1998. "Medicaid program; Medicaid managed care; proposed rule." *Federal Register* 63 (September 29th): 52021–52092.

Kilborn, P. T. 1998. "Complaints about H.M.O.'s rise as awareness grows." *New York Times* (October 11th): 22.

Pear, R. 1998a. "Administration to set down new protections for H.M.O. Medicaid patients." *New York Times* (September 17th): A24.

Pear, R. 1998b. "Senators reject bill to regulate care by H.M.O.'s." *New York Times* (October 10th): A1, A10.

Trafford, A. 1998. "The hidden heart of an HMO." *Washington Post Health* (May 12th): 6.

10

Some Unresolved Issues

The differences between those who are disvalued because they are disabled and the nondisabled are narrowing, not because of changes in attitudes, but because of a vast change in how we pay for and organize health care in the United States. This might be called a harsh version of the democratic ethos of the country, since we are all in this together. People with disabilities are facing the same transition to managed care as those without disabilities. The traditional American fee-for-service system, with its multiplicity of choices for those with indemnity coverage, is being rapidly converted into managed care systems, with all the features discussed in chapter 3. This enormous social and economic transition intensifies concerns for people with serious physical and mental health conditions because lack of access to optimal medical care can involve serious risks to life and endanger the quality of their lives.

The emphasis on cost containment, it appears, produces grave consequences for those who are heavy users of the health care system. The emphasis on primary care and prevention, the use of primary care providers as gatekeepers to specialists and hospital admission, and the limited access to specialists has, in the past, created disincentives for people with disabilities to join managed care plans. Alternatively, people with disabilities have recognized the value of greater care coordination, ease of access to primary care providers, and the elimination of substantial deductibles and substantial percentages of the charges or co-payments that makes managed care attractive to those with disproportionate usage of the health care system.

While the public, in general, has been satisfied with the quality of health care received from MCOs, there has been a great deal of worry and uncertainty expressed in opinion polls. This suggests that there is a generalized concern among survey respondents, and if they are a representative sample, a similar concern among all Americans, about what will happen to them when faced with a serious chronic illness or disability. Will quality care be accessible to them when they are really in need of complex interventions and not merely routine care? The questions that are asked are called, in the public opinion survey trade, "hypotheticals," revealing that the answers are not based on direct experiences. Yet there is enough information from our friends, neighbors, relatives, and co-workers to put a scare into us, that is, the American public, about whether managed care will truly be there when we face a health crisis.

The Association of Health Plans and some of the defenders of managed care in the survey research industry (Ladd, 1998) suggest that the longer people are in an MCO, the higher the level of satisfaction. While it is true that it takes some time to adjust to the rules found in MCOs, there is also another factor that confounds this result, and flagrantly flaws any argument that the happy member is the one who has stayed a long time in the plan. What happens to people who are deeply unhappy with their health plan? They drop out, or, as labor leaders say when workers conduct wildcat strikes, "they vote with their feet." The argument can be made that the most dissatisfied are not being polled because they are not in plans, or after joining another plan, are not asked about their experience with the first plan, the one that they left.

The transition to managed care has also created new priorities for providers as well as for patients. Since it is the medical profession that uses up resources and is the actual consumer of health care, particularly the big-ticket items, for example, hip replacement, its members are the target of efforts by managed care plans to stay within a fixed budget. Gone are the days when the patient was seen as a serviceable or repairable object and everything was done that might work. Now the patient in need of fixing is seen as a "cost center," a burden that the medical practice has to bear.

The philosophy of practice today is to care for the entire panel of patients rather than the individual. Consequently, needy individuals may not receive optimal care. Capitation as a form of payment to a medical group or to an individual provider encourages the idea of providing "minimally acceptable" care, a management concept that attempts to rein in the extravagant providers who do everything for a patient. Naturally, to create even more uniformity within the health care corral, the providers are given incentives in the form of withholds and bonuses for husbanding scarce resources (Kassirer, 1998). Finally, it may be that the care you get is the care you are entitled to, as when providers carefully tailor procedures performed to the package of procedures allowed by the plan.

For every doctor who seeks to practice according to an older style of focusing on what needs to be done, there may be three doctors willing to work under the new regime. The profession does not have the solidarity today to refuse to participate in MCOs that promote: suboptimal care; nondisclosure of financial incentives; and heavy expenditures on advertising, stock options for executives, and high stockholders' profits. Doctors who have opted out of managed care often cater to the very wealthy who can afford indemnity insurance (usually provided as a benefit), with high deductibles and co-payments. One wonders whether the chief executive officers of HMOs and other managed care organizations have benefits similar to those of most middle-class Americans, or if their health insurance policies allow them to opt out of the health care revolution, as so many of the wealthy are able to do.

Not withstanding the prior comments, there is still some merit in the argument that providers should pay attention to the entire patient panel, particularly since wellness care does have substantial payoffs for patients. The attentiveness to the entire panel should also involve creating policies that encourage the identification of enrollees who are functionally disabled and live in the community. They should not fall between the cracks in the system, to resurrect an old cliché. This is particularly important for plans that attract large numbers of Medicaid- and Medicare-eligible individuals, who often have severe disabilities that qualify them for those public insurance programs. Given their ticket into managed care, their plans need to assess all newcomers for disability, and refer to case management or care coordination services those individuals who require greater medical attention.

Referral is not enough. Programs of care coordination need to be in place in publicly funded MCOs and those with private insurance support. The goal of care coordination should not be to save money but rather to maintain or improve the functional status and independence of people with disabilities, as stated in "Standards and guidelines for review of Medicare and Medicaid managed care organizations" (National Academy for State Health Policy, 1997). Optimal programs of this kind, through interventions, seek to slow the rate of decline in functional status, particularly among elderly patients. Furthermore, there is good reason to be flexible with this segment of the covered lives in an MCO. Where appropriate, specialists should be allowed to be the primary care providers.

Enrolling large numbers of people with disabilities may also involve making physicians' offices wheelchair accessible. When HMOs were simply staffed medical centers where a large number of physicians were to be found, it was cost-effective to remodel the facility to meet the Americans with Disabilities Act's requirements. Now HMOs and other managed care organizations are built around a network of physicians and other health care providers who are dispersed all over a metropolitan region in offices with varying accessibility to people with mobility limitations. This is not a mere theoretical possibility, because as more and more people with these type of impairments have to use new providers in accordance with their plan, it will become more evident that plans are not set up to accommodate them. What this means is that persons with disabilities may not be as free to choose a provider from within the plan as other members might. According to the barriers found, and many older buildings still have them, they may have to choose on the basis of the availability of a ramp or elevator.

The goals of integration and inclusion are not always in line with the revolution in health care. For the disabled in a five-county area in and around Philadelphia, the name of the plan HealthChoices may have a hollow ring to it. In the U.S. District Court for the Eastern District of Pennsylvania, a judge ruled that all of the 5,200 doctors and dentists in the Philadelphia metropolitan area who participated in the state-funded managed care program, HealthChoices, must have offices that are accessible to people with mobility impairments. Following inspection by the Department of Public Welfare, any provider who did not eliminate barriers to people with mobility impairments would be terminated from the state's new HMO Medical Assistance Program. In addition, within 60 days of signing an agreement between the Disabled in Action of Pennsylvania, the plaintiffs in the suit, and the department, there must be available, upon request by HealthChoices members, informational materials about the plan in Braille, large print, and on audiocassette tape (Disability News Service, 1998: 4).

This is not the complete list of accommodations needed for people with disabilities when it comes to accessing medical services. There may be a need for medical transportation for those with mobility limitations, interpreter services for the deaf, special examining tables, and also personal assistance services for the severely physically impaired. None of these services is mentioned in the marketing of managed care plans, perhaps because the plans do not want to attract people with disabilities. Nevertheless, even individuals who are medically stable but have functional deficits will need some of these forms of enabling services.

Managed care plans are cost-aversive, meaning that what appears to the managers of these plans to be disproportionately expensive may become highlighted and a cause for concern. Early interventions that may be expensive but are also cost-effective in the long run may not get done because the member may not belong to the plan 10 years from the time of the performance of procedures, or are not done because they are ruled not therapeutic.

MANAGED CARE AND PEOPLE WITH DISABILITIES

Once inside the friendly confines of managed care, what kinds of uncertainties can people with disabilities anticipate? First, the gatekeeping function of primary care providers especially reveals some of the conflicts that occur in the payer, provider, patient triangle. In the past, the physician was a trusted protector of the interest of the patient and was not implicitly asked to balance the needs of the patient against the needs of the corporate entity that contracted for the physician's services. Some advocates for people with disabilities argue that the various risk-sharing arrangements that are there to make the physician sensitive to using tests and making referrals to specialists should not be allowed as a source of remuneration for physicians. Therefore, the gatekeeper should not be put in the position of having to choose between obligations to patients and financial incentives, or obligations to employer or payer for services. Financial incentives that encourage restraint in the delivery of services may mean that access to care is limited arbitrarily.

There is special concern on the part of the critics of managed care that unless clinical practice guidelines are closely followed there is some likelihood that a serious condition will be misdiagnosed as a minor illness, or that it will be overlooked entirely. This increase in the incidence of what is known as "false negatives"—the diagnosis of no disease being present when it actually is present—is a great concern. There have been a number of cases leading to litigation where precisely this type of error has occurred in HMOs and where patients have died or suffered the serious consequence of not receiving treatment for something that can be treated.

Reduced access to specialty care implies that it is precisely this kind of error that will increase when managed care becomes even more prevalent than it is. Whereas past errors in medical diagnosis were likely to be "false positives," or identifying a disease being present when it actually was not there, the newer restraints on practice hardly encourage such outcomes. Litigation that follows misdiagnoses with harmful results always involves the physician—and if the plan is making medical decisions through prior authorization requirements—it should involve the plan as well.

Access to specialists who can provide optimal care is as important to a plan member as access to early detection of disease. Any health plan will overtly enumerate in detail its benefits and limits when attempting to recruit individual consumers. Less explicit are the methods of restricting providers in such ways that consumers cannot learn how their access to service is limited. These limits can be harmless or full of consequences for consumers. Members are within their rights in demanding to know how their health plan's contracts with physicians impinge on their care and information about their care.

Optimal care should not be excluded from the plan because of the provider recruitment patterns. Sometimes a patient has a very rare condition that is best treated by an expert specialist who may not be a member of the plan. When a plan promises to provide all the medical care required, that means that even if patients come down with conditions that the HMO doctors are unfamiliar with, they still have to make state-of-the-art medical care available. Consumers want to know that a plan can actually say that it went the "extra mile" for a patient and delivered what was needed—not that it refused to pay for a consultation with a physician who was not a plan participant. This kind of pre-emptive refusal to seek the best medical care possible is similar to health insurers dropping enrollees who are making claims for covered services related to catastrophic illnesses.

There is also sometimes an implicit restriction of access to needed care that is not known to the patient. A clear decision cannot be made by patients when physicians restrict or withhold information. Most controversial are the previously discussed "gag clauses," contract wording that forbids doctors from working for the patient in need. These restrictions interfere with the basic trust that must be established between doctor and patient.

The health plan should include support for patients with regard to all the medical problems encountered, not just approved treatments. With interventions the subject of evaluation, there is a need to determine if they work and patients actually benefit from the procedures performed. This kind of inquiry seeks greater accountability. Thus, an attempt could be made to see if HMOs do a better job than fee-for-service indemnity coverage policies in keeping people well or curing them.

In order to make such comparisons, as well as comparisons between HMOs, data collection must include large enough samples so that age, severity of the disease, and other variables can be held constant. Employers who purchase group coverage through HMOs are becoming more and more concerned about quality benchmarks that go beyond signing up board-certified providers and high rates of immunization and screening (e.g., mammography).

The question remains, do these interventions make a difference? While a cure rate is difficult to measure, it is possible to compare how well health plans are able to reduce cholesterol levels and hypertension, or prevent individuals from being hospitalized for decubitus ulcers. These kind of interventions have to do with the active management of disability rather than a simple follow-up of screening. An even better gauge of effectiveness, claims disability activist Ray Seltser, is an improvement in the level of functioning or a return to normal activity.

The development of such measures of accountability are particularly important as Congress encourages Medicaid- and Medicare-eligible individuals to join HMOs. HMOs that specialize in these populations will be under the closest scrutiny because the various encouragements offered individuals with a disproportionate number of impairments will raise new questions about the quality of care under managed care. The development of these new outcome measures is good for health care in general but they come at a price. The shift to managed care has created more interest in quality measurement than in the past, and also makes these health plans spend more time and money justifying their existence. Health service research has now become a growth industry in the age of managed care.

In the past, this branch of research has made some extraordinary discoveries, full of policy implications. One of the great discoveries of these investigators was that when it came to doing complex procedures, there were differences in outcomes according to how frequently those interventions were performed. Thus, with regard to cardiac arterial bypass grafting, there were some surgeons who had better outcomes than others, even when researchers controlled for the degree of severity of the damage to the patients' hearts and circulatory systems that brought them in to face the knife.

Given the success of these busy surgeons, sick patients sought them out, and they developed a great deal of experience in treating this population. Experience seemed to count and be rewarded in the old fee-for-service system, and thoracic surgeons who took on the most difficult cases were admired. In the world of managed care the successful surgeons may avoid the most critically ill because they increase the likelihood that they will have to spend more time with patients, order more tests, and prepare to operate.

A similar pattern may emerge with HMOs or medical groups that contract with managed care plans that have extraordinary success in medical management of disabilities. They can develop reputations that they can ill-afford to have. How can our health care system continue to reward the pursuit of excellence when it comes to medical practice—and therefore encourage physicians and surgeons to gain experience working with the most difficult cases when the new managed care reward system is organized around risk avoidance?

HEALTH CARE AS A PUBLIC UTILITY

It is useful to make some comparisons with our neighbors to the north to better understand what drives financing and decisions about whether the entire population should be covered by health insurance. Moreover, it also puts care for people with disabilities, because of their vulnerability under managed care, on the top of the agenda when it comes to correcting the system. Disproportionate users of the health care system need to gain access to quality care but they are often the targets of cost containment efforts. How can they be protected from medical neglect and also contribute their fair share to cost containment?

The American health care system is financed by public and private contributions, with management of the actual providers in the hands of private ownership. Any proposed reform or change in the health care system shakes individual doctors who own their own practices as well as for-profit hospital chains, and multistate managed care organizations. These interests have a great deal—in the way of financial resources—at stake, will spend a lot to protect their financial interests, and consequently, will fight legislation that threatens regulation or promotion of public ownership of the means to deliver health care in the United States. In addition, a substantial part of the cost of care in the United States is paid for by employers in the private sector.

In contrast, in Canada, the recognition that health care is in both private and public hands, but financed almost completely from public funds raised through taxes, has created (or results from) a sense of social solidarity among all its citizens. Canadians believe that health care is a right of all, and there are no uninsured in Canada. The concerns of the business interests are much less a part of the way budgeting occurs for this necessary service than in the United States where employers who contribute to the system have made their views much more prominent when it comes to determining how to spend that money.

Increasingly health care is becoming privately collectivized through the growth of managed care in the United States. Profits are made when health care expenditures are kept lower than the MCO's dollar intake. Known as the medical-loss ratio, this figure is used by profit-making HMOs to lure investors. However, health care is not simply a commodity that is bought and sold according to market rates. Affordable health care and optimal care are needed for all citizens. Consider this analogy: State commissions regulate power suppliers so that rates for consumers are kept reasonable. To make managed care work better, HMOs must also be held responsible for what they do in a public way. Government oversight is necessary to ensure that patients get the care they need. A public utility is regulated for the benefit of all citizens. Bob Griss (1997: 4) clearly points to the incompatibility of the need for increased capacity to provide care for all with private owner-ship and profits for stockholders. The public utility focus is necessary to equalize access to quality care and to ensure that all public resource alloca-tion decisions are made not only on the basis of changes in the health status of enrollees in a specific managed care plan, but also on the basis of changes in the health status of the total population. This broader context is critical because the profit-maximizing strategies within the corporate economy of a specific health plan may strengthen or undermine society's capacity to ef-ficiently serve the total population (4).

THE REPORT CARD

The designers of evaluation and accountability for HMOs have pro-moted their quality assurance efforts so that consumers will be able to com-fortably join a plan, knowing that the plan they join has been accredited by the National Committee on Quality Assurance. However, people with dis-abilities are left out of this marketing process in several ways.

First, they are few in number compared to the far larger number of people in an HMO without disabilities, and the conditions that they must deal with cannot be aggregated sufficiently so that statistical tests can be per-formed. Second, because their conditions are less prevalent, there has been less effort made by providers both outside and inside of managed care to develop clinical practice guidelines. Therefore, it is not possible to deter-mine whether state-of-the-art practices were undertaken in a particular MCO. Nor are outcomes measurable in the form of fewer days missed from work or school.

A serious movement in the direction of quality assurance and quality improvement needs to occur among providers of care for people with dis-abilities so that plans can be rewarded for keeping people well or optimizing their functional potential.

This brings us back to those "centers of excellence" in the disability field, which can increase the capacity of MCOs to care for people with dis-abilities. In order to be a useful resource to MCOs, centers of excellence must be given incentives to continue to develop and test new program ap-proaches, to create innovations in applying diagnostic techniques and interventions, to conduct research to determine what works and what does not, and to identify what is cost-effective. More and more evidence-based decisions about future treatments will be required and these centers will have to have a role in providing that evidence. Therefore, they should have an important role in the development of practice guidelines and quality assurance measures. Finally, they must continue research and related dissemination efforts to assure that new approaches are tested and new knowledge is disseminated, including information about how new technology can be utilized. Obviously, the use of the Internet and distance-learning techniques (including possible use of self-study programs by care providers) may be applied. Wherever possible, university-affiliated programs (UAPs) and other "centers of excellence" must provide technical assistance to elected policy makers, government officials, and HMO leadership to promote appropriate practices and care provisions.

"CENTERS OF EXCELLENCE" INTEGRATED IN MANAGED CARE ORGANIZATIONS[1]

Since considerable specialized expertise exists at academic medical centers, both in medical and allied health disciplines, and since those programs also have extensive experience in developing and utilizing interdisciplinary service models, they can provide certain specialized services to clients served in managed care systems.

There are cultural differences between academic medical centers and MCOs. Unfortunately, managed care systems are accustomed to a single consultation model wherein they refer a patient to one specialty provider for his or her opinion and require that the primary care physician be the source of the referral and the recipient of the consultant's views. While UAPs, for example, may be in a position to provide a single consultation through a developmental pediatrician, pediatric neurologist, physiatrist, psychiatrist, geneticist, or other specialist, the usual UAP model is to initiate an interdisciplinary team evaluation using a selection of medical and allied health specialists. These may range from a psychologist, social worker, speech pathologist, and special educator to additional professionals such as a nutritionist, occupational therapist, physical therapist, audiologist, and others. This evaluation tends to be more costly than the single consultation model.

Furthermore, the traditional HMO may be accustomed to using a "mental health" contractor to provide any "psychological" services, while a developmental disability service provider usually offers psychological assessments, psychometric testing, and/or behavioral management in a program that does not consider itself, or wish to be labeled, a "mental health" center or program.

What then can or should be the service role of centers of excellence in the world of managed care? A key role is in diagnosis and assessment that will help the individual, the family, and the primary care physician understand the nature of the individual's disability, establish a medical diagnosis where applicable, determine the child's or adult's functional level, and, if required, help determine the individual's eligibility for educational, income, or vocational training entitlement programs. In serving in the latter capacity, these highly specialized clinical programs can be one of the "gatekeepers," assisting local, state or federal agencies in making eligibility determinations by supplying accurate information about the child's or adult's needs. The center's clinical expertise also may assist the HMO in determining the patient's legitimate need for other specialized services, therapies, durable medical equipment, specialized transportation, medications, and so forth.

One may ask, why should the HMO want this information, if it may cost them more to provide for their patient's special needs? Putting aside the serious ethical or legal questions associated with possible rationing of care, as well as the HMO's need to sustain its reputation as a quality service provider, there are some cost-saving benefits of the subspecialist involvement. These may include: (1) help in determining patients' eligibility for government entitlement programs that will reduce the HMO's need to pay for certain services; and (2) providing the expertise that may help the HMO differentiate between an evidence-based, useful treatment methodology and an unorthodox or inappropriate, costly intervention that some less experienced or less scientifically knowledgeable providers may recommend. Experience has shown that many unnecessary or excessive therapies may be prescribed by non-university based providers, interventions that more knowledgeable academic-based professionals may not support.

Also important is the role of skilled professionals in early identification of a developmental disability that may not only lead to a referral to the early intervention and special education systems in each state, but also to interventions that may reduce the long-term costs of care. A good example is the role that early physical therapy plays to prevent contractures in children with cerebral palsy, thereby reducing the need for later costly hospitalizations and surgery.

However, to fulfill a useful role for an MCO, the highly specialized clinical program will have to modify its approach. No longer can the expensive interdisciplinary evaluation be used for all referrals. Some programs already screen each referral, either in person or by telephone, and then attempt to make an initial determination of how a case should be processed. In some cases, a single consultation will be initially offered and then a decision can be made about whether additional consultations or tests are required. In other cases, a smaller interdisciplinary team can be assembled, with only specific required specialists participating so that the evaluation will be limited to the aspects of the problem that there are clear needs to define. In other cases, where a more extensive evaluation may be required, shared evaluation visits using groups of professionals may expedite evaluations, avoid duplication, and result in reduced costs.

In other cases, skilled case management can be provided to HMO clients that will facilitate the evaluation process and improve coordination among team members, as well as with the referring physician or other care providers in the HMO. Case management and care coordination are certainly other important components that subspecialty care providers at centers of excellence can offer to HMO patients.

The training role of centers of excellence in relation to the evolving managed care systems has not been clearly defined. One major problem identified by consumer groups is that many primary care providers, both in HMOs and outside of these systems, lack the clinical skills, knowledge, communication skills, attitudes, and sensitivity to appropriately manage the care for individuals with disabilities and help their families or care givers.

There are two possible approaches to rectify the problem. The first is to introduce the issues to physicians-in-training, beginning when they are medical students and then during their residency training, so that they may have a significant exposure to the diagnosis and treatment of children and adults with developmental disabilities. Thus far, only board-certification requirements in pediatrics demand at least a one-month training experience in developmental and behavioral pediatrics. This usually includes a rotation to a developmental clinic serving children with disabilities and/or related chronic illnesses. In most instances, center-operated clinics and their faculty serve that training role in the teaching hospitals and medical centers where they are based.

The second approach to improving training is through continuing education of physicians currently enrolled in provider organizations and/or nurse practitioners and others serving HMOs as primary care providers. This would require that programs like the UAPs reach out to HMO care providers and administrators to assure the availability of satisfactory continuing education experiences. This can only be achieved if there is pressure from consumer groups and other advocacy organizations to force

HMO leadership to require the participation of their primary care providers, as well as their care coordinators and other decision makers.

Briefly, this training should deal with how to identify disabilities early; when and how to make appropriate referrals for interdisciplinary diagnosis and treatment; and ways to enhance knowledge about available community resources, provide reliable information about the prognosis and the anticipated life cycle of individuals with different types and degrees of disabilities, and impart a clear understanding of families' needs, largely through consumer input.

To reach this level of partnership between MCOs and centers of excellence requires a strategy for making these programs the sole-source providers of the training and services described in the previous paragraphs. How can this be accomplished?

A STRATEGY FOR SOCIAL MARKETING

Despite my recommendation that MCOs be regulated as public utilities, there still need to be efforts made to get these plans to provide optimal care based on existing resources. Where in the past the strategy might only be to develop public policy recommendations to enable people with disabilities to receive appropriate services, the challenge today is also to develop appropriate *marketing strategies* to reach the private and public purchasers of services. As in other disciplines, there may be nothing more practical than a utopian vision, not only of the future state of medical care, but of a strategy for preserving the best of contemporary practice.

Many medical center- and university-based services are recognized in their communities as the "benchmark" for services to children, adolescents, and adults—both with and without disabilities. It seems ironic that to continue to maintain high-quality services, the academic medical centers and their subspecialty centers must demonstrate their value.

The idea of marketing services and overall capability is no stranger to these academic medical centers. Many of the new mergers among medical schools and academic medical centers in the East (e.g., New York Presbyterian) create marketing strategies to keep their specialties busy. An effective marketing strategy will help to make the future more predictable for centers of excellence and involves adjustments to a changing social and economic environment.

Subspecialty care providers can add value to their work and help the new financing and delivery systems provide better services if they can convince MCOs to see them as partners and even "internal" suppliers of something that they need. The goal of such a strategy is that the centers of excellence become providers of clinical services, training, technical assistance and dissemination of research and information about developmental disabilities to managed care organizations and health maintenance organizations.

The guidance for this strategy is derived from customer- driven social marketing (Andreason, 1995). This concept is largely the result of efforts to change behavior to promote health, social development, and the environment. There is no reason why it cannot be applied to changing the behavior of MCOs.

Unlike other kinds of marketing, in social marketing customers are listened to carefully to determine how the future will be better for the target audience. In addition, various groups of people are heard from in a similar way. Therefore, to develop an appropriate marketing strategy, not only are organizational decision makers studied through the needs and wants of the purchasers of these services (benefits managers/employers, HCFA), but also through the requirements of the consumers (work-derived group plan enrollees, mandatory Medicaid managed care recipients, Medicare recipients).

Owing to the strong commitment of MCOs and HMOs to continuous quality improvement, market research should be aimed at determining to what extent the following efforts have been undertaken to promote better health outcomes for people with disabilities:

- implementation of needs assessments of all new enrollees;
- assuring that correct diagnoses are made;
- adoption or creation of clinical practice guidelines for low prevalence conditions;
- use of care coordination/case management;
- permitting specialists to serve as primary care providers (PCPs) under special circumstances;
- special recruitment or training of some or all PCPs to create internal capacity for providing appropriate medical services for people with disabilities; and
- evidence of the development of outcome measures for treatment for low prevalence conditions.

One way to implement this social marketing research is to randomly select a sample of 100 corporate members of the American Association of Health Plans (AAHP) and to submit a self-administered survey based on these quality improvement measures. The goal is to determine if optimal care is in place for people with disabilities. Other survey items related to organizational characteristics will help to determine which types of arrangements predict high use of these quality improvement efforts. In addition, data has to be collected about the standard metropolitan statistical areas (SMSA) that these plans serve to determine whether demographic characteristics predict use of these quality improvement measures. Finally, the market characteristics of these SMSAs (e.g., mature markets, high HMO or MCO penetration) must be determined.

After analyzing the data from the survey, face-to-face interviews must be conducted with the major decision makers at MCOs and HMOs to determine their attitudes, beliefs, knowledge and behavioral responses regarding (1) disabilities and (2) the use of academic-based agencies such as UAPs for providing health services, training, and knowledge. What do they perceive as the benefits and costs of providing services for people with developmental disabilities? What do they perceive as the importance of these services to purchasers of their plan's coverage or to the actual users of the plan's services? Are there any social pressures on them to create partnerships with academic medical centers?

Following data collection, analysts need to determine what are the major impediments to the proposed partnerships with UAPs. What factors in the internal environments of MCOs and HMOs and in the external environment (e.g., public opinion, state and federal regulation) would influence them to change their behavior with regard to centers of excellence?

Social marketing attempts to understand customer behavior and how it changes could be accomplished by using the following heuristic device. Customers are seen as being in one of four possible stages of adoption of the appropriate behavior: precontemplation stage, contemplation stage, action stage, or maintenance stage. Communications depend then on which stage the customer is determined to be at. For example, there is some evidence to suggest that MCO and HMO executives may not know how many members have disabilities of any kind. At such a stage (precontemplation), the message might be geared to let the decision makers know that there is interest in finding out how people with disabilities fare in these plans. Information from benefits managers or the executives' significant others (e.g., relatives and friends or family members with developmental disabilities) will create a potential positive reward for them to pay attention to continuous quality improvement mechanisms that can benefit health plans and their enrollees. To wit, it may be in the MCO's interest to provide optimal care, not just consider the medical-loss ratio. Plans that have a surplus at the end of the year might consider sharing it with enrollees.

Not all executives will respond equally well to the same message. Segmentation of the market is a prime consideration. Communications should not be the same for different levels of management. Some may be concerned more with future returns on investments, while those with medical backgrounds may be under cross-pressure from their corporation and their profession. Physicians and other health care providers often resent the recent and rapid collectivizing of the health care industry under large for-profit corporations and their new "double agent" status: Is their loyalty to the health plan or as a medical care provider, to the patient?

The social transformation of health care during the past decade through the growth of MCOs has meant that for physicians and other health care providers the profit motive is now a major distraction from delivery of quality patient care. A mechanism for refocusing professional energies is called for. There may be a need to create a newsletter for these role players that focuses on managed care (as a delivery system) and developmental disabilities. Consciousness raising would be attempted in the first three issues as concerns over access and quality are brought to the forefront by analysts and advocates (e.g., Bob Griss from the Center on Disability and Health).

Later issues would include guest articles from friendly executives from MCOs and HMOs that talk about the cost-offsets produced by some of the quality improvement milestones developed in cooperation with centers of excellence. Of course, this product and others should come out of newly established marketing divisions at appropriate national organizations.

These associations could, for example, present an award, similar to the Malcolm Baldridge award for excellence, to the HMO or MCO that has done the most to provide quality services for people with disabilities. It would be useful to put together a distinguished committee to review applicants for this award and to alert the media to what is happening. The committee, of course, should include consumers and family members as well as professionals. One quality to look for is extensive partnering with quality service providers.

It will be very important to advertise the existence of this award in the appropriate journals and Internet venues. In anticipation of criticism, I could see where one might object to establishing an award because no health plan might apply. If that is the case, the media should be apprised of this fact. If there are deserving MCOs and HMOs, this should be brought to the attention of the membership of the AAHP, particularly to those that find it too costly to partner with a center of excellence or introduce the previously mentioned quality improvement measures. The prize winner should become the benchmark for the industry and this prize should be awarded for at least 10 years. When MCOs and HMOs seek to become more efficient in the delivery of services for people with disabilities, all efforts at continuous quality improvement will be based on this role model. Perhaps in the future there will be no need for the award because the distinguished panel would not be able to distinguish between best practices of MCOs and HMOs since they would all be at the same level of excellence.

Structuring

After approving the basic strategy and a detailed plan, an organization or team has to be put in place to carry out the core strategy as stated above. The plan should be rewritten at this point in time to achieve a level of specificity previously uncaptured. Following the methodology of Walter Shewart (1931), an early inventor of quality control in industry, that was adopted by health care providers to ensure quality improvement, we need to Plan-Do-Check-Act.

The following steps are necessary: (1) key elements of the program deemed worthy should be pretested before full implementation is attempted; and (2) monitoring of the progress of implementation needs to be ongoing and not just a part of a final evaluation. According to advocates of social marketing, micromanaging of the program usually involves changes in midcourse, with adjustments in strategy and tactics as needed. Most important, the customers are still being listened to even at the late stages of the program.

A sound strategy that promotes a sustainable plan will provide a vision for the future for both the customers and the sponsors of the plan. It should provide a sense of security for the UAPs and a sense of fairness for the MCOs and HMOs. The elements should be clearly conveyed to the team and the target audience, creating a viable partnership. Finally, the marketing strategy should be open to change should unforeseen contingencies arise.

Despite the capacity of disability advocates, centers of excellence, and enrollees to develop a plan for integrating into the new managed care health system, the industry itself needs to be made more of a partner with providers and consumers, rather than a controlling force for cost containment. Regulating an industry that impacts on millions of covered lives seems to be in order. Yet once again in 1998, as in 1994 during the halcyon days of health care reform, there were campaign funds being garnered from the health insurance industry to effectively kill off a Patient Protection Act or a Patient Bill of Rights Act. Once again, the Republican motto was "Don't just do something, stand there!" While this legislation is likely to return to the national agenda, there is little hope of a public debate in the Senate, let alone passage of a bill, as long as campaign finance reform remains a dream. Americans continue to let their elected officials stretch out their hands and lower their eyes when funds are being passed around.

NOTE

1. This section is based on excerpts from Herbert J. Cohen and Arnold Birenbaum, "Managed care and quality health services for people with developmental disabilities: Is there a future for UAPs?" *Mental Retardation* (August 1998): 325–329. Used by permission of AAMR.

REFERENCES

Andreason, A. R. 1995. *Marketing Social Change: Changing Behavior to Promote Health, Social Development, and the Environment.* San Francisco: Jossey-Bass Publishers.

Disability News Service. 1998. "Mandatory managed care programs must provide accessible providers." *Disability News Service's E-News* (August): 4.

Griss, R. 1997. "People with disabilities and managed care: A litmus test for cross-subsidization, quality assurance and consumer empowerment." *Maximizing Human Potential* 5 (Summer): 1–4.

Kassirer, J. P. 1998. "Managed Care—should we adopt a new ethic?" *New England Journal of Medicine* (August 6th): 339.

Ladd, E. C. 1998. "Health care hysteria, part II." *New York Times* (July 23rd): A25.

National Academy for State Health Policy. 1997. "Standards and guidelines for review of Medicare and Medicaid managed care organizations." Unpublished paper. Portland, ME: National Academy for State Health Policy.

Shewart, W. 1986. *Economic Control of Quality of Manufactured Product.* Milwaukee: ASOC Quality Press. (Original work published 1931)

Further Reading

Disability and Managed Care joins the issues and is derived from a diverse set of publications and Internet sources. As a book, it may stand by itself, for the moment, as we move into the new millennium. There are now many books on managed care or health maintenance organizations, but they rarely deal with disability. In addition, there are numerous recent books about the personal experience of disability. However, I suspect that in the next few years we will not see either subject rival the number of confessional style volumes by the Clintons, Henry Hyde, Monica Lewinsky, and Linda Tripp. Still this mess had a disability angle: It was gratifying to see Charles Ruff, an exceptional lawyer and a wheelchair user, lead the charge in the Senate trial against removing the president from office.

My preceding remarks about America's recent trials and tribulations are not fully gratuitous. The backdrop of this work is the effort by the first Clinton administration at reforming our health care system. That failure opened the door to the market-driven reforms that have focused mostly on reducing costs and little on increasing access to or quality of care. These reforms have created new dangers and opportunities for people with disabilities in the world of health care.

My concern for recent data, sophisticated policy analyses, and systematic health services research made me rely on many articles and editorials from *The New England Journal of Medicine*, *The Journal of the American Medical Association*, and *Health Affairs*. In particular, the continuously fine work on the changing financing of the health care system by John K. Iglehart in the *New England Journal of Medicine* stands out. Not to be left behind, during the past decade, even more narrowly focused journals—such as *Mental Retardation*—included some thoughtful policy analyses of the implications of managed care for people who cannot fully take care of themselves. For further reading, timely and impartial studies on controversial aspects of health care were done by the Congressional Budget Office and the United States Government Accounting Office.

Managed care was also a story with "strong legs," as journalists say. The national press was always there for me. Newspapers that have public policy commitments are often way ahead of the reviewed journals. They were very helpful in dealing with late-breaking policy questions, details on the business-end of health maintenance organizations, and how consumers are responding to managed care. My home-delivered *New York Times* often made me late for work as I attempted to read lengthy articles about our changing health care system. I am especially indebted to the excellent analysis and reporting by Robert Pear and Milton Freudenheim. I read less systematically in the *Washington Post* and the *Wall Street Journal*, two daily papers that also keep up with the revolution in managed care. The weekly news and business magazines, in their consumer-friendly ways, also had stories about the best and worst in HMOs. A more solid source of rating health plans was the monthly magazine *Consumer Reports*. For the past 15 years, this nonprofit independent publication has been involved in broadly analyzing the growth of managed care, how its readership responded, and how to make it work.

One of the major public debates emerging in the future—given consumer outrage about managed care—will be concerned with how much government regulation should take place in the health care marketplace. Troyen A. Brennan and Donald M. Berwick's *New Rules: Regulation, Markets, and the Quality of American Health Care* (1996) is a brilliant effort that argues forcefully that a strong emphasis on quality management and outcomes research can reduce sharply the need for consumer protection.

But can this heady view win the day? As my son Jonathan used to say, I doubt it. As I write, Congress, in its effort to grab onto a small-bore populist issue, is seeking to create consumer protection in this era of managed care, and simultaneously, to promote memory loss over the recent impeachment and trial of President Clinton. Readers will do well to turn to the Web site of *Families—USA* for detailed side-by-side analyses of prospective legislation from the perspective of individuals with specific medical needs and whether the different bills would afford them protection. Again on the Web, the Robert Wood Johnson Foundation's home page can leader the reader to systematic studies of the impact of managed care on services for people with serious chronic illnesses and disabilities.

To understand things fully from a disability advocate's perspective, including the implications of pending legislation, or lack thereof, I would read the tightly written broadsheets available from the Center on Disability and Health, 1522 K St., Suite 800, Washington, D.C. 20005. Bob Griss, the center's director, and major policy analyst, is also a master of the spoken word and would do well generating talking books.

Index

About the Author

ARNOLD BIRENBAUM is Associate Director, University Affiliated Program, Department of Pediatrics, Albert Einstein College of Medicine. Professor Birenbaum has written extensively on health and public policy issues, including *Putting Health Care on the National Agenda* (Greenwood, 1995) and *Managed Care: Made in America* (Greenwood, 1997).